GASTROENTEROLOGY
QUICK GLANCE

GASTROENTEROLOGY QUICK GLANCE

Z. Colette Edwards, MD, MBA

Vice President and Senior Market Medical Executive
CIGNA HealthCare
Cleveland, Ohio

McGraw-Hill
MEDICAL PUBLISHING DIVISION

New York / Chicago / San / Francisco / Lisbon / London / Madrid / Mexico City
Milan / New Delhi / San Juan / Seoul / Singapore / Sydney / Toronto

The **McGraw·Hill** Companies

Gastroenterology Quick Glance

1 2 3 4 5 6 7 8 9 0 DOC/DOC   0 9 8 7 6 5

ISBN: 0-07-142190-4

This book was set in Palatino by Silverchair Science + Communications, Inc.
The editors were James Shanahan, Karen G. Edmonson and Penny Linskey.
The production supervisor was Catherine H. Saggese.
The book designer was Marsha Cohen.
The cover designer was Aimee Nordin.
The indexer was Pamela Edwards.
RR Donnelley was printer and binder.

This book is printed on acid-free paper.

Cataloging-in-Publication data for this title is on file with the Library of Congress.

"I am only one, but still I am one. I cannot do everything, but still I can do something. And because I cannot do everything, I will not refuse to do the something that I can do."

Edward Everett Hale

This book is dedicated to Drs. Mattie, Zeno, and Tanise Edwards who paved the way to make one of my dreams come true.

C O N T E N T S

Contributors / ix
Abbreviation Legend / xi
Preface / xv

GASTROINTESTINAL TRACT / 1

1	Diarrhea Syndromes	3
2	Motility Disorder Syndromes	25
3	Intestinal Ischemia Syndromes	35
4	Polyposis and Colon Cancer Syndromes	43
5	Inflammatory Bowel Disease	53
6	Gastrointestinal Genetics Pearls	63
7	Gastrointestinal Bleeding	69
8	Diverticular Disease	75

THE LIVER AND BILIARY TREE / 79

9	Hepatitides	81
10	Autoimmune Liver Disease	101
11	The Porphyrias	109
12	Hepatology Drug Review	117
13	Genetic Liver Disease	123
14	Surgical Considerations	129
15	Miscellaneous Hepatology Pearls	135

Benign Recurrent Intrahepatic Cholestasis / 135
Work-Up of Ascites / 135

Portal Gastropathy/Colopathy / 137

Varices / 137

Hepatorenal Syndrome (HRS) / 137

Hepatopulmonary Syndrome / 138

Acute/Fulminant Hepatic Failure / 138

Orthotopic Liver Transplantation (OLT) / 138

Cancer / 139

16   The Biliary Tree   145

THE PANCREAS / 151

17   The Pancreas   153

MULTISYSTEM DISORDERS / 167

18   Endocrine Syndromes   169

19   Pregnancy Syndromes   175

20   Clinical Nutrition   179

21   Nutritional/Vitamin Deficiency and Toxicity Syndromes   193

22   Acquired Immune Deficiency Syndrome (AIDS)   205

RELATED TOPICS / 211

23   Dermatologic Manifestations of Gastrointestinal   213
     and Liver Disease

24   Radiologic Imaging of the Gastrointestinal Tract,   217
     the Liver, and Biliary Tree

25   Pathology of the Gastrointestinal Tract, Liver,   227
     and Biliary Tree

26   Bariatric Surgery   235

27   Gastrointestinal Malignancy Surveillance Protocols   241

28   Miscellaneous Clinical Pearls   247

QUICK GLANCE REVIEW GRIDS / 251

29   Quick Glance Review Grids   253

Index / 313

Hobart W. Harris, MD, MPH

Professor and Chief
Division of General Surgery
Department of Surgery
University of California, San Francisco
San Francisco, California

Chapter 5, Chapter 14, Chapter 16, Chapter 17, Chapter 26

Antoinette Saddler, MD

Assistant Professor, Internal Medicine
Digestive Health Centers of Excellence
Division of Gastroenterology and Hepatology
University of Virginia Health System
Charlottesville, Virginia

Chapter 20

Michael T. Schell, MD

Research Fellow
Department of Surgery
University of California, San Francisco
Surgical Research Laboratory
San Francisco, California

Chapter 5, Chapter 14, Chapter 16, Chapter 17, Chapter 26

ABBREVIATION LEGEND

A

Ab = antibody
abd = abdomen, abdominal
abx = antibiotics
ACE = angiotensin converting enzyme
Addn'l = additional
AIDS = acquired immune deficiency syndrome
ALT = alanine aminotransferase
AP (view) = antero-posterior
AST = aspartate aminotransferase
avg = average

B

BI = Billroth I
BII = Billroth II
BAO = basal acid output
BCP = birth control pills
bili = bilirubin
BMs = bowel movements
BMT = bone marrow transplant
bx = biopsy

C

Ca = cancer
CBD = common bile duct
CEA = carcinoembryonic antigen
CHD = common hepatic duct
CHF = congestive heart failure
Cipro = ciprofloxacin
CLD = chronic liver disease
CMV = *Cytomegalovirus*
CNS = central nervous system
CREST = *c*alcinosis, *R*aynaud's syndrome, *e*sophageal dysmotility, *s*clerodactyly, and *t*elangiectasia
CRI = chronic renal insufficiency
CRF = chronic renal failure
CSF = cerebrospinal fluid
cx = culture

D

DC-BE = double-contrast barium enema
DDx = differential diagnosis
DIC = disseminated intravascular coagulopathy
DM = diabetes mellitus
DU = duodenal ulcer
DVT = deep vein thrombosis
dx = diagnosis
dz = disease

E

Echo = echocardiogram
EGD = esophagogastroduodenoscopy
Endo = endoscopy, endoscopic
Eos = eosinophils
ERCP = endoscopic retrograde cholangio-pancreatography
ESLD = end-stage liver disease

esoph = esophagus, esophageal
ETOH = alcohol (ethanol)
ETOHA = alcohol abuse
EUS = endoscopic ultrasound
EVL = endoscopic vein ligation
extrem = extremity/extremities

F

FNH = focal nodular hyperplasia
FOBT = fecal occult blood test
F/U = follow-up
fx = fracture

G

GAD = gadolinium
GAVE = gastric antral vascular ectasia
GB = gallbladder
GI = gastrointestinal
GIB = gastrointestinal bleed
GOO = gastric outlet obstruction

H

HA = headache
HCC = hepatocellular carcinoma
HDL = high-density lipoprotein
h/o = history of
HSV = *Herpes simplex virus*
HTN = hypertension

I

IBD = inflammatory bowel disease
IBS = irritable bowel syndrome
IC = ileo-cecal
IVF = intravenous fluids

L

L = left
LCHAD = long-chain 3 hydroxyacyl CoA dehydrogenase
LDH = lactate dehydrogenase
LES = lower esophageal sphincter
LESP = lower esophageal sphincter pressure
LFTs = liver function tests
LLQ = left lower quadrant

M

MAC = *Mycobacterium avium complex*
MALT = mucosa-associated lymphoid tissue
MMCs = migratory motor complexes
MRA = magnetic resonance angiography
MRCP = magnetic resonance cholangio-pancreatography

N

NASH = nonalcoholic steato-hepatitis
neuro = neurologic, neurological
NTG = nitroglycerin
N&V = nausea and vomiting

O

osteo = osteomyelitis
OLT = orthotopic liver transplant

P

path = pathology
PBC = primary biliary cirrhosis
PCN = penicillin
PD = pancreatic duct
PE = pulmonary embolism

plt(s) = platelet(s)
PMNs = polymorphonuclear leukocytes
PPIs = proton pump inhibitors
prn = as needed
prodn = production
prods = products
PSC = primary sclerosing cholangitis
PT = prothrombin
pts = patients

R

R = right
RBCs = red blood cells
RNA = ribonucleic acid
r/o = rule out
RTA = renal tubular acidosis
RUQ = right upper quadrant
Rx = medication

S

SBFT = small bowel follow-through
SBO = small bowel obstruction
SBP = spontaneous bacterial peritonitis
SLE = systemic lupus erythematosus
sx = symptoms
sz = seizure

T

TB = tuberculosis
TCN = tetracycline
TG = triglycerides
TI = terminal ileum

TIPS = transjugular intrahepatic porto-systemic shunt
TMP-SMX = trimethoprim-sulfamethoxazole
TP = total protein
TPN = total parenteral nutrition
TNTC = too numerous to count
TTP = thrombotic thrombocytopenic purpura
tx = treatment, therapy

U

U/A = urinalysis
UDCA = ursodeoxycholic acid
UGI = upper GI
U/S = ultrasound

V

VIP = vasoactive intestinal peptide
vit = vitamin

W

WBCs = white blood cells

X

XRT = radiation therapy

MISCELLANEOUS

$\Rightarrow$ = implies, indicates, suggests
$\rightarrow$ = leads to, results
$\uparrow$ = increase/increased, elevated
$\downarrow$ = decrease/decreased, reduction
+ = plus, positive

This book began as a collection of tables I designed for myself to be used as summary study guides on a select range of topics in preparation for the gastroenterology recertification exams. The original format has been retained in adjunctive exhibits in the last chapter, but the remaining content has been translated to a more traditional format, and the topic list has been expanded.

The intended audience of this text includes, but is not limited to, practitioners in medicine ranging from medical and nursing students to actively practicing clinicians in all specialties who find a need for a succinct overview reference of key topical areas in the field of gastroenterology. For those studying for gastroenterology certification and recertification exams, the original intent remains just as applicable as when the first study grids were designed.

The text is divided into 6 sections – the gastrointestinal tract, the liver and biliary tree, the pancreas, multi-system disorders, related topics, and quick glance review grids – with chapters that cover a broad range of subjects in the field of gastroenterology, hepatology, and gastrointestinal surgery. A PDA program is also available.

To close, I will leave you with the following thoughts which I believe serve clinicians (and their patients) well in both their studies and the care they provide:

".... One of the most helpful maneuvers.... is to listen carefully to the patient, who will often provide the answers needed to make an accurate diagnosis. Failure to heed a patient's words may needlessly delay an evaluation or result in inappropriate treatment and/or unnecessary testing."

Z. Colette Edwards, MD
Gastroenterology. *Urgent Care Medicine* (editors Edwards & Mayer)
New York; McGraw-Hill, April 2002:327 – 354.

".... In order to provide safe and optimal care...., it is important in approaching each patient .... to recognize what one knows, recognize what one doesn't know, and care enough about the patients to seek consultation whenever needed."

Tanise I. Edwards, MD
Preface. *Urgent Care Medicine* (editors Edwards & Mayer)
New York; McGraw-Hill, April 2002: xii.

PART I

GASTROINTESTINAL TRACT

CHAPTER 1

DIARRHEA SYNDROMES

DIARRHEA SYNDROMES
Highlights

► **Helpful in differentiating syndromes:**
  • gender
  • symptoms and demographics
  • lab profile
► **Major Syndromes - Bacteria:**
  • *Vibrio cholerae*
  • non-cholera vibrio (parahaemolyticus)
  • *Escherichia coli*
  • *Listeria*
  • *Staphylococcus aureus*
  • *Bacillus cereus*
  • *Campylobacter jejuni*
  • *Salmonella*
  • *Shigella*
  • *Yersinia*
  • *Clostridium difficile*
  • *Clostridium botulinum*
  • *Clostridium perfringens*
  • *Aeromonas*
  • *Plesiomonas*
  • tuberculosis
  • tropical sprue
  • *Tropheryma whippelii* (Whipple's disease)
► **Major Syndromes - Viruses:**
  • *Rotavirus*
  • Norwalk agent

- CMV
- HSV
- Additional Pathogens: Adenovirus, Astrovirus, Calicivirus
► **Major Syndromes - Parasites:**
  - *Giardia lamblia*
  - *Cryptosporidia*
  - *Microsporidia*
  - *Isospora belli*
  - *Cyclospora cayetanensis*
  - *Entamoeba histolytica*
  - Miscellaneous Parasitic Agents:
    - *Entamoeba coli*
    - *Entamoeba hartmanni*
    - *Endolimax nana*
    - *Iodamoeba buetschlii*
    - *Blastocystis hominis*
    - *Balantidium coli*

General Information

► 9 L fluid/day - 8 L absorbed in small bowel and 1 L absorbed in colon
► absorption - primarily via villi
► secretion - primarily via crypts
► diarrhea - decreased absorption and/or increased secretion
► The greater the number of polys, the lower in the GI tract the problem originates.
► sheets of polys $\Rightarrow$ colonic problem
► small bowel - large volume, watery, diffuse crampy abd pain, malabsorption, dehydration
► large bowel - small volume, frequent BMs, lower abd pain, dehydration
► inflammatory - frequent mucoid and/or bloody stools, may be accompanied by tenesmus, fever, severe abd pain + fecal WBCs and frequently occult blood
► noninflammatory - watery stools, frequently large volume, without blood or WBCs, absence of abd pain and fever
► infectious - acute onset, fever early, > 4–6 BMs/day, short duration of illness (24–48 hours), normal architecture on path
► IBD - fever uncommon, chronic, insidious onset, < 4–6 BMs/day, abnormal crypt architecture

TABLE 1-1
OVERVIEW OF DIARRHEA

Features	Secretory	Osmotic	Comments
Osmotic gap: 290 − [Na+ + K+] × 2	< 20	> 30	
Fecal osmolality	280 − 400 mOsm/L	260 − 300 mOsm/L	Normal = 260 − 280 mOsm/L
Volume	Large	< 1 L/d	
Impact of fasting	Persists	Decreases	
Stool pH	< 6.0	< 7.0	
Causes	1. Infection & bacterial enterotoxin	1. Poorly absorbed solutes (e.g., magnesium, antacids, sorbitol, mannitol, phosphate)	
	2. Neurohumoral agents (e.g., VIP, serotonin, calcitonin, gastrin, prostaglandins)	2. Maldigestion (e.g., pancreatic insufficiency, disaccharidase deficiency)	
	3. Detergents (e.g., bile salts, fatty acids as seen in TI resection)	3. Malabsorptive disorders (e.g., mucosal defects, bacterial overgrowth)	
	4. Laxatives		

▶ bile salt - voluminous, burning, occurs with eating
▶ diabetic diarrhea:
  • occurs in 1–5% of diabetics (usually type I with autonomic neuropathy and end-organ damage)
  • variable clinical course - unpredictable, episodic, may alternate with constipation (constipation more common complaint in diabetics than diarrhea), may be nocturnal/ urgent/accompanied by incontinence/large volume
  • correlates poorly with state of glycemia
  • most common cause - metformin
  • 25% may have steatorrhea
  • need to R/O celiac sprue, pancreatic insufficiency, bacterial overgrowth

▶ microscopic colitis:
  • sx: secretory, watery, weight loss, abrupt onset, 60–70 yo
  • dx: flex with at least 5 bx
  • bx: intraepithelial lymphs
  • can co-exist with celiac sprue
  • frequently abates within 2 years
  • tx: loperamide/Lomotil → bismuth → 5-ASAs → cipro/metronidazole → steroids → 6-MP/azathioprine
▶ DDx of "chronic traveler's diarrhea" - unmasked IBD, postinfectious IBS, celiac sprue, persistent infection (*Giardia*, amebiasis, *Salmonella, Campylobacter, Yersinia*), *C. difficile*, lactose intolerance, tropical sprue, bacterial overgrowth
▶ bacterial overgrowth (blind loop syndrome) - diarrhea-steatorrhea (due to bile salt deconjugation) + macrocytic anemia (due to vit B_{12} deficiency); may also see hypoalbuminemia; abx tx: cipro + metronidazole × 7 days; may need repeat/cyclic/prolonged courses
▶ 4 most common pathogens implicated in bloody diarrhea in U.S.:
  1. *Campylobacter*
  2. *Salmonella*
  3. *Shigella*
  4. *E. coli O157:H7*
▶ infectious:
  • small bowel: usually noninvasive, viruses most frequent pathogens
  • large bowel: likely invasive, bacteria most frequent pathogens
  • parasites typically noninvasive and fungi extremely uncommon cause in immunocompetent individual
▶ indications for treatment in infectious diarrhea:
  • suspected shigellosis or toxic appearance (e.g., moderate to severe diarrhea, > 6 BMs/d, high fever)
  • severe enteritis
  • traveler's diarrhea
  • immunosuppression
▶ specific pathogens which should be treated:
  • *Shigella*
  • *C. difficile*
  • *Yersinia*
  • *Campylobacter*
  • non-cholera vibrio

- sexually transmitted pathogens
- prolonged sx: *Aeromonas, Plesiomonas,* enteropathogenic *E. coli*
► antibiotics for empiric therapy:
  - quinolones (but not in children): drug of choice for entero-pathogenic, enterotoxigenic, *Shigella,* cholera
  - TMP-SMX
► specific parasitic clinical syndromes:
  - malabsorption: *Giardia, Strongyloides,* coccidiosis, *Cryptosporidia, Isospora belli, Capillariasis*
  - bloody diarrhea: amebiasis, schistosomiasis, trichuriasis
  - occult blood in stool: hookworm, *Strongyloides*
  - chronic tropical diarrhea: **bacteria** - *Salmonella*; **parasites** - ameba, post-amebic dysentery, *Giardia,* coccidiosis, *Cryptosporidia, Isospora belli*; tropical sprue
► string test - *Giardia,* coccidiosis, *Strongyloides*
► Scotch tape test - enterobiasis (pinworm)
► ascaris (hookworm; a nematode in the helminth family) - #1 parasite worldwide
► ingestion of preformed toxins (e.g., *S. aureus, Bacillus cereus*) - sx within 6 hours
► incubation of 8–12 hours ⇒ *C. perfringens*
► incubation > 14 hours ⇒ viral or invasive pathogen

Demographics
Bacteria
► ***Vibrio cholera*** - diarrhea due to toxin disruption of cAMP and prodn of PLT-activating factor; incubation: hours - 7 days; endemic in southern Asia, Africa, Latin America; source: seafood, fecally contaminated water; at risk: primarily children, pregnant women, hypochlorhydria, immunosuppressed; primary infection associated with immunity for at least 3 years
► **Non-cholera vibrio (parahaemolyticus)** - associated with undercooked seafood, eggs, potatoes, exposure to dogs
► ***E. coli*** - 5 species:
  - 3 species affect small bowel via enterotoxin:
    1. enteroadherent
    2. enteropathogenic (EPEC)
    3. enterotoxigenic (ETEC)
  - ETEC: frequent cause of traveler's diarrhea
  - transmission: contaminated food or water

TABLE 1-2
CAUSES OF ACUTE DIARRHEA

Noninflammatory diarrhea[a]	Inflammatory diarrhea[b]
Viral	**Viral**
Norwalk virus	Cytomegalovirus[c]
Rotavirus	**Bacterial**
Protozoa	**1. Cytotoxin production**
Giardia lamblia	*E. coli* O157:H7
Cryptosporidium	(enterohemorrhagic)
Bacterial	*Vibrio parahaemolyticus*
1. Preformed enterotoxin	*Clostridium difficile*
Staphylococcus aureus	**2. Mucosal invasion**
Bacillus cereus	*Shigella*
Clostridium perfringens	*Salmonella sp.*
2. Intraintestinal enterotoxin	Enteroinvasive *E. coli*
production	*Aeromonal*
E. coli (enterotoxigenic)	*Yersinia enterocolitica*
Vibrio cholerae	*Plesimonal*
New medications	**3. Bacterial proctitis**
Fecal impaction	*Chlamydia*
	N. gonorrhoeae
	Protozoal
	Entamoeba histolytica
	Intestinal ischemia
	Inflammatory bowel disease
	Radiation colitis

[a]Noninflammatory: Fever absent. Stool without evidence of blood or fecal leukocytes.
[b]Inflammatory diarrhea: Often with systemic features, including fever. Fecal leukocytes with or without gross blood usually present. (**Note:** Fecal leukocytes are variable in *Salmonella, Yersinia, V. parahaemolyticus, C. difficile,* and *Aeromonas*.)
[c]Most commonly in immunocompromised patients, especially AIDS.

- 2 species affect colon:
  1. enteroinvasive (EIEC)
  2. enterohemorrhagic (EHEC)
- EHEC: *E. coli* O157:H7; source: unpasteurized dairy, undercooked beef, fecally contaminated water; produces 2 *Shigella*-like toxins; sx often localized to R side of colon, therefore may mimic ischemic colitis in elderly and intussusception or IBD in pediatric population; causes 10% of cases of acute diarrhea and has < 1% overall mortality rate

▶ *S. aureus* - 2nd most common cause of bacterial food poisoning; produces at least 7 enterotoxins; full recovery within 48 hours; attack rate of 80–100%; Gram-positive coccus

TABLE 1-3
CAUSES OF CHRONIC DIARRHEA

Osmotic diarrhea
  Lactose intolerance
  Medications: sorbitol, lactulose, antacids
  Factitious: magnesium laxatives or sodium sulfate laxatives
  Clues: Stool volume decreases with fasting; increased osmotic gap
  > 50 mOsm/L
Malabsorptive conditions
  Intestinal mucosal diseases: celiac sprue, Whipple's disease,
  eosinophilic gastroenteritis, Crohn's disease, small bowel
  resection
  Lymphatic obstruction
  Pancreatic disease: chronic pancreatitis, pancreatic carcinoma
  Small bowel bacterial overgrowth: motility disorders (vagotomy,
  scleroderma, diabetes), colonic-enteric fistulas, small intestinal
  diverticula
  Clues: Weight loss, fecal fat > 7–10 g/24 h stool collection, anemia,
  hypoalbuminemia
Secretory diarrhea
  Hormonal secretion: VIPoma, carcinoid, medullary carcinoma of
  thyroid, Zollinger-Ellison syndrome (gastrinoma)
  Bile salt malabsorption: ileal resection, Crohn's disease
  Medications
  Factitious: phenolphthalein, cascara, senna
  Villous adenoma
  Clues: Large volume (> 1 L/d); little change with fasting (except
  with bile salt diarrhea); normal stool osmotic gap
Inflammatory conditions
  Ulcerative colitis
  Crohn's disease
  Microscopic colitis
  Radiation enteritis
  Malignancy: lymphoma, adenocarcinoma
  Clues: Fever, hematochezia or abdominal pain (absent in
  microscopic colitis)
Motility disorders
  Postsurgical: vagotomy, partial gastrectomy
  Systemic disorders: scleroderma, diabetes mellitus,
  hyperthyroidism
  Irritable bowel syndrome

▶ *Bacillus cereus* - Gram-positive rod; 5th most common cause of
  food poisoning; produces toxin; resolution of sx within 48 hours
▶ *Campylobacter jejuni* - transmission via oral-fecal route or contaminated milk, poultry, eggs, water

TABLE 1-4
CLINICAL FEATURES ASSISTING IN THE DIFFERENTIATION OF A SMALL BOWEL FROM
COLONIC DIARRHEA[a]

Feature	Small intestine	Colon
Stool frequency	Frequent	Frequent
Stool volume	Large	Small
Stool character	Watery	May be bloody
Electrolyte abnormalities	+++	—
Dehydration	++	—
Weight loss	+	+
Abdominal pain	+	++
Borborygmi	+	—
Upper GI tract symptoms	+	—
Fecal leukocytes	Absent	Present with colitis

[a]+++, very common; ++, frequent; +, can occur; —, not seen.

▶ **Salmonella** - 2200 serotypes of *Salmonella*; carrier state if stools positive at 1 year
  • *Typhi* (typhoid fever):
    ▪ fecal-oral contamination → food transmission: poultry, eggs, dairy, water; gallbladder reservoir
    ▪ incidence: infants, elderly
    ▪ increased risk: achlorhydria, sickle cell, chronic schistosomiasis, ETOH, cardiovascular dz
  • *Gastroenteritis/enterocolitis* (nontyphoidal):
    ▪ transmission: contaminated animal products (eggs, turkey, meat, milk)
    ▪ high-risk: < 5 yo, homosexual men, DM, sickle cell, malaria, institutionalized
▶ *Shigella* - 4 species: dysenteriae, flexneri, boydii, sonnei; colitis caused by invading colonic epithelium and by producing enterotoxin; most common in 1–4 yo, homosexual men, travelers, institutionalized; transmission: fecal-oral via contaminated hands
▶ *Yersinia* - uncommon in U.S.; common in Northern Europe; source: contaminated milk or pork via fecal-oral route
▶ *C. difficile* - most common nosocomial infection of GI tract; more common with po abx
▶ *C. botulinum* - produces neurotoxin that blocks acetylcholine; source: improperly canned foods, raw honey
▶ *C. perfringens* - produces enterotoxin; source: improperly stored beef, fish, poultry, pasta salads, dairy products, Mexican food; recovery usually within 24 hours

TABLE 1-5
INFLAMMATORY AND NONINFLAMMATORY DIARRHEA

	Inflammatory diarrhea	Noninflammatory diarrhea
Clinical presentation	Small-volume, bloody diarrhea; lower abdominal cramping or pain; fecal urgency; tenesmus; sometimes, fever	Large-volume, watery diarrhea; upper or paraumbilical abdominal pain or cramping; possible nausea or vomiting
Presence of fecal leukocytes	Yes	No
Common causes	*Shigella, Campylobacter, Salmonella, E. histolytica, Yersinia,* enteroinvasive *E. coli, C. difficile*	*Vibrio, Giardia, Cryptosporidia,* enterotoxigenic *E. coli,* rotavirus, Norwalk virus, toxigenic food poisoning (*S. aureus, C. perfringens, B. cereus*)

TABLE 1-6
COMPARISON OF BILE ACID AND FATTY ACID DIARRHEA

	Bile acid diarrhea	Fatty acid diarrhea
Extent of ileal disease	Limited	Extensive
Ileal bile acid absorption	Reduced	Reduced
Fecal bile acid excretion	Increased	Increased
Fecal bile acid loss compensated by hepatic synthesis	Yes	No
Bile acid pool size	Normal	Reduced
Intraduodenal (bile acid)	Normal	Reduced
Steatorrhea	None or mild	>20 g
Response to cholestyramine	Yes	No
Response to low-fat diet	No	Yes

▶ *Aeromonas* - source: contaminated water or shellfish; often seen in children

▶ *Plesiomonas* - source: contaminated water or shellfish; often seen in children

▶ **Tropical sprue** - usually seen in residents or long-term visitors (> 1 year) in Africa, Middle East, Cuba, Central America, Puerto Rico, Haiti, Dominican Republic; results from persistent contamination of small bowel with toxigenic strains of coliform bacilli with overgrowth of *Klebsiella, E. coli, Enterobacter cloacae*

TABLE 1-7
AGENTS IMPLICATED IN DRUG-INDUCED DIARRHEA (ACCORDING TO PATHOPHYSIOLOGIC MECHANISMS)[a]

Secretory
  Antineoplastics
  Auranofin (gold salt)
  Calcitonin
  Cardiac glycosides
  Colchicine
  Nonsteroidal antiinflammatory medications
  Prostaglandins (misoprostol)
  Stimulant laxatives (bisacodyl, phenolphthalein)
  Ticlopidine
Osmotic
  Laxatives and sugar-free products (lactulose, sorbitol, fructose, mannitol)
  Magnesium (laxatives, antacids)
  Secondary to maldigestion of carbohydrates
    Antibacterials (ampicillin)
    Acarbose (α-glucosidase inhibitor)
Motility
  Colchicine
  Macrolides (erythromycin)
  Thyroid hormones
  Ticlopidine
Exudative
  Antineoplastics
  Nonsteroidal antiinflammatory medications
  HMG-CoA reductase inhibitors (i.e., simvastatin)
  Ticlopidine
Fat malabsorption
  Aminoglycosides
  Auranofin (gold salt)
  Biguanides
  Cholestyramine
  Colchicine
  Laxatives
  Methyldopa
  Octreotide
  Polymyxin, bacitracin
  Tetracyclines

[a]Modified from Chassany O, Michaux A, Bergmann JF. Drug-induced diarrhea. *Drug Safety* 2000;22:53.

in most; distinguished from classic small bowel overgrowth by presence of only 1–2 species
► *Tropheryma whippelii* (**Whipple's disease**) - most cases: 50 yo white males; 25% HLA-B27

Viruses
► **Rotavirus** - RNA virus; 48–72-hour incubation; fecal-oral, person-to-person transmission; incidence greatest in children 6–24 months old; 80–100% of children have Ab by age 2
► **Norwalk agent** - source: contaminated water and shellfish; fecal-oral, person-to-person, and airborne transmission; 24–48-hour incubation
► **CMV** - seen in immunocompromised
► **HSV** - sexually transmitted
► **Additional pathogens** - Adenovirus, Astrovirus, Calicivirus

Parasites
► *Giardia lamblia* - transmitted by ingestion of contaminated food and water or via fecal-oral contact; 5% of traveler's diarrhea; common in freshwater streams and lakes and in the western U.S. and eastern Europe
► *Cryptosporidia* - CD4 often < 100; mainly found in the jejunum and ileum
► *Microsporidia* - prevalence of 10–30% in AIDS; CD4 usually < 50
► *Isospora belli* - incubation of 7–11 days; outbreaks in day care centers and mental health institutions
► *Cyclospora cayetanensis* - transmission via fecal-oral contact or drinking contaminated water; outbreaks associated with raspberries, basil
► *Entamoeba histolytica* - transmission via fecal-oral route; colonizes 10% of world's population but only results in symptoms in 10% of cases

Symptoms/Signs/Labs

Bacteria
► *Vibrio cholera* - epidemic cholera, vomiting, metabolic acidosis, altered sensorium, sz, electrolyte imbalance, death markers: ileus, arrhythmias, muscle cramps
► **Non-cholera vibrio (parahaemolyticus)** - self-limited diarrheal illness: dysentery, N&V, HA, fever
► *E. coli:*
   I. Small bowel:
      • self-limited watery diarrhea
      • EPEC (enteropathogenic): watery diarrhea, vomiting, fever; usually seen in infants

- EIEC (enteroinvasive): fever, malaise, watery diarrhea with blood or mucus, cramps; may see fecal RBC and WBC
- ETEC (enterotoxigenic): traveler's diarrhea

II. Colon:
- EHEC (enterohemorrhagic) clinical syndromes:
  a. hemorrhagic colitis
  b. hemolytic uremic syndrome (hemolytic anemia, DIC, renal failure)
  c. nonbloody diarrhea

▶ EHEC - watery diarrhea and cramps followed by bloody diarrhea 12–24 hours later, fever and vomiting in < 25%, sx 1–2 weeks (with shedding of organism 4–8 weeks); complications: hemolytic uremic syndrome (in 2–7% with a 10% mortality rate), TTP, most common in children or those with severe bleeding and WBC > 20K

▶ *S. aureus* - N&V and cramps followed by diarrhea

▶ *Bacillus cereus*
- fried rice → vomiting, cramping
- meat, vanilla sauce, salad, chicken soup, cream-filled baked goods → profuse watery diarrhea, cramping

▶ *Campylobacter jejuni* - sx 1–7 days after ingestion; nausea, anorexia, cramping, watery or bloody diarrhea; can mimic appendicitis; colitis frequent; Guillain-Barré syndrome frequent sequelae

▶ *Salmonella*
- Typhi (typhoid fever): prolonged fever, abd pain, diarrhea, GIB, rose spots, splenomegaly, possible perforation; resolution of sx after 4 weeks
- gastroenteritis/enterocolitis (nontyphoidal) presentations:
  - asxtic carrier
  - acute gastroenteritis/colitis/ileocolitis
  - enteric fever with bradycardia, rose spots, splenomegaly, leukopenia
  - bacteremia dysentery uncommon
  - self-limited illness
  - extraintestinal complications: osteo, mycotic aneurysm, meningitis

▶ *Shigella* - toxin: small bowel, watery diarrhea; invasion: colon with dysentery; begins in small bowel with fever, nausea, cramps, and secretory diarrhea followed by localization in colon with resultant ulcers and inflammation, bloody mucoid diarrhea and tenesmus, systemic toxicity; may see toxic mega-colon and obstruction; mortality rate of 9%, usually in children < 9 yo and usually due to dehydration; extraintestinal compli-cations: hemolytic uremic syndrome, pneumonia, sz, encepha-lopathy, malnutrition, Reiter's syndrome (triad of arthritis, ure-thritis, conjunctivitis): most common in men 20–40 yo, seen 2–4 weeks after infection, predilection for HLA-B27

▶ *Yersinia* - diarrheal syndrome; can mimic appendicitis or Crohn's disease when presents as acute terminal ileitis; can cause acute or chronic colitis; postinfectious complications - erythema nodosum, polyarthritis in HLA-B27, Reiter's syndrome

▶ *C. difficile* - fever, abd pain, diarrhea with gross or occult blood; may develop toxic colitis/megacolon; 12–24% recur-rence rate; risk factors for recurrence: old age, intercurrent abx, renal dz, prior recurrences; 2–8% mortality rate with toxic megacolon

▶ *C. botulinum* - mild nausea, vomiting, diarrhea, abd pain, neuro sx: diplopia, ophthalmoplegia, dysarthria, dysphagia, dysphonia, descending weakness, paralysis, respiratory muscle paralysis; may take months to recover

▶ *C. perfringens* - watery diarrhea, cramping without vomiting; may see necrotizing enterocolitis

▶ *Aeromonas* - self-limited watery diarrhea with blood and mucus; extraintestinal manifestations - sepsis, meningitis, endophthalmi-tis, arthritis, cellulitis, cholecystitis

▶ *Plesiomonas* - self-limited watery diarrhea with blood and mucus; extraintestinal manifestations - sepsis, meningitis, endophthalmitis, arthritis, cellulitis, cholecystitis

▶ **Tropical sprue** - acute watery diarrhea with cramping and gas which becomes chronic; lactose and ETOH intolerance, folate defi-ciency within 2–4 months → anorexia, weight loss and folate and B_{12} deficiency within 6 months → megaloblastic anemia with weakness and glossitis; may also see ↓ carotene, vit A, vit D, albu-min, cholesterol, calcium

▶ *Tropheryma whippelii* (**Whipple's disease**) - weight loss up to > 100 lbs, diarrhea, arthralgias (migratory, large joints, precedes dx by 9 years, attacks lasting hours to days, sacroiliitis in 20–30%), fever, abd pain, occult GIB, pericarditis and endocarditis in 50–75%, systolic murmur in 25%, peripheral lymphadenopathy in 50%, oculomasticatory myorhythmia unique to Whipple's; CNS - dementia, personality change, Wernicke's disease, ataxia; anemia - chronic disease, folate and B_{12} deficiency, $\downarrow$ albumin, $\uparrow$ PT, abnormal D-xylose in 80%; weight loss, diarrhea, fever precedes dx 1–4 years

Viruses
▶ **Rotavirus** - severe diarrhea, vomiting, profound dehydration, metabolic acidosis, electrolyte disturbance, low-grade fever, pharyngitis, otitis media
▶ **Norwalk agent** - diarrhea with N&V, low-grade fever, cramping, myalgias, anorexia, HA
▶ **CMV** - self-limited colitis
▶ **HSV** - distal proctitis following anal intercourse, severe anal pain and discharge, urinary retention, pain in abdomen/buttocks/thighs
▶ **Miscellaneous Pathogens** - Adenovirus, Astrovirus, Calicivirus

Parasites
▶ *Giardia lamblia* - crampy abd pain, nausea, bloating, flatulence, anorexia, explosive watery, foul-smelling, greasy diarrhea; chronic infection in immunoglobulin deficiency
▶ *Cryptosporidia* - profuse, watery diarrhea, vomiting, crampy, abd pain, flatulence, weight loss, afebrile, malabsorption, B_{12} deficiency, lactose intolerance
▶ *Microsporidia* - multiple, watery BMs, abd discomfort with flatulence, weight loss with good appetite, afebrile, malabsorption
▶ *Isospora belli* - hemorrhagic ulcerative colitis
▶ *Cyclospora cayetanensis* - prolonged, watery diarrhea (4–6 weeks) usually without fever, prodrome of flulike illness and profound fatigue and GERD may overshadow diarrheal illness
▶ *Entamoeba histolytica* - range of sx: asxtic carrier state - severe dysentery, hepatic abscess; colicky abd pain, diarrhea alternating with constipation, may get toxic megacolon, may mimic colon ca with strictures/amebomas on DC-BE
▶ Additional agents - *Entamoeba coli, Entamoeba hartmanni, Endolimax nana, Iodamoeba buetschlii, Blastocystis hominis, Balantidium coli*

Diagnosis

Bacteria
▶ *Vibrio cholera* - stool cx

▶ **Non-cholera vibrio (parahaemolyticus)** - stool cx with selective culture techniques

▶ *E. coli* - stool cx with serotyping of Ag; EHEC dx: stool cx on sorbitol-MacConkey agar, ELISA- cytotoxin in stool, colonoscopy with bx useful

▶ *S. aureus* - clinical scenario, cx

▶ *Bacillus cereus* - clinical scenario

▶ *Campylobacter jejuni* - stool cx

▶ *Salmonella* - stool cx

▶ *Shigella* - stool cx; may see positive blood cx in AIDS

▶ *Yersinia* - stool cx with special cold-enrichment technique; can also cx lymph nodes, blood, peritoneal fluid but takes weeks; serology with elevated antibody titers; colonoscopy - aphthoid ulcers, round/oval elevations of mucosa

▶ *C. difficile* - stool cx

▶ *C. botulinum* - detection of toxin in stool or vomitus

▶ *C. perfringens* - demonstration of organisms in food or stool

▶ *Aeromonas* - stool cx

▶ *Plesiomonas* - stool cx

▶ **Tuberculosis** - colonoscopy with bx for histologic diagnosis or microbiologic confirmation with acid-fast stain; may see strictures, deformed ICV, ulceration; may mimic Crohn's or colon ca

▶ **Tropical sprue**:
1. ↓ D-xylose absorption
2. steatorrhea in 50–90%
3. abnormal glucose tolerance test in 50%
4. thickened and coarsened mucosal folds on small bowel barium study
5. bx: broadening and shortening of villi, infiltration of lamina propria with chronic inflammatory cells

▶ *Tropheryma whippelii (Whipple's disease)* – PAS-positive bacilli in macrophages on small bowel bx (need 4–6 bx; take bx for electron microscopic evaluation as well)

Viruses

▶ **Rotavirus** - stool antibody assay

▶ **Norwalk agent** - no commercially available diagnostic tests

▶ **CMV** - biopsy

▶ **HSV** - viral isolation from culture of rectal swab or bx; flex sig helpful: focal ulcers and vesicles

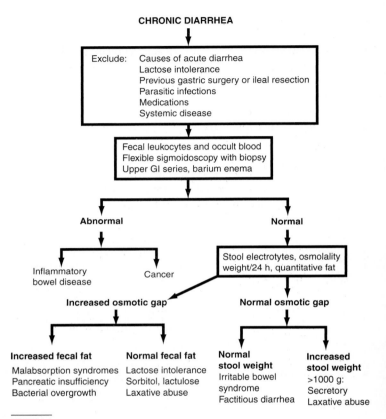

FIGURE 1-1

Diagram for diagnosing causes of chronic diarrhea. (Reproduced with permission from Friedman SL, McQuaid KR, Grendell JH, *Current Diagnosis & Treatment in Gastroenterology*. Lange Medical Books/McGraw-Hill, 2003.)

Parasites

▶ *Giardia lamblia* - cysts in stool (need 3 stools over 6 days due to intermittent excretion); duodenal aspiration for trophozoites; *Giardia* antigen

▶ *Cryptosporidia* - acid-fast or immunofluorescent monoclonal antibody stain of stool

▶ *Microsporidia* - trichrome or Weber's chromotrope-based stain of stool followed by confirmatory fluorescence staining

- ► *Isospora belli* - duodenal aspirate/biopsies, diagnosis by stool exam difficult
- ► *Cyclospora cayetanensis* - positive acid-fast or safranin stain
- ► *Entamoeba histolytica* - check stool or swab for cysts/trophozoites

Treatment

Bacteria
- ► *Vibrio cholera* - Options:
    1. TCN
    2. chloramphenicol
    3. TMP-SMX
    4. ampicillin
- ► **Non-cholera vibrio (parahaemolyticus)** - TCN in severe infection
- ► *E. coli* - Options:
    1. TMP-SMX
    2. cipro
- ► Anti-motility agents decrease sx.
- ► EHEC - antibiotics not recommended; may increase toxin production
- ► *S. aureus* - rehydration
- ► *Bacillus cereus* - fluid resuscitation and anti-emetics
- ► *Campylobacter jejuni* - treatment recommended for severe enteritis lasting longer than 1 week
- ► Options:
    1. erythro
    2. TCN
    3. cipro
- ► *Salmonella*
    - typhi: tx not recommended as it prolongs excretion and increases relapse rate; if necessary, cipro or TMP-SMX
    - nontyphoidal: indicated in severe sx, very young, elderly, pregnant women, immunocompromised, severe underlying illness; rx: chloramphenicol, high-dose ampicillin or amoxicillin, TMP-SMX, cipro, ceftriaxone
    - carrier state: quinolones
- ► *Shigella* - tx shortens duration of sx and decreases excretion of pathogens

- Options:
    1. ampicillin
    2. TMP-SMX
    3. nalidixic acid
    4. cipro × 5 days - drug of choice
- *Yersinia* - tx recommended in severe enteritis, mesenteric adenitis, erythema nodosum, and arthritis
- Options:
    1. TCN
    2. TMP-SMX
    3. chloramphenicol
    4. cipro
- *Clostridium difficile* - should avoid anti-diarrheals - Options:
    I. Diarrheal syndrome:
        a. first line - metronidazole 250 mg po qid × 10 days
        b. vancomycin 125 mg po qid × 10 days
    II. Toxic megacolon:
        a. metronidazole 500 mg IV q 6–8 hours
        b. to consider:
            ■ IV vanco
            ■ colonoscopic decompression
            ■ cecostomy
        c. surgical resection prn
    III. Recurrent diarrheal syndrome:
        a. repeat course of same or alternative abx
        b. cholestyramine or colestipol
        c. *Saccharomyces boulardii*
        d. *Lactobacillus*
- *C. botulinum* - antitoxin, supportive care
- *C. perfringens* - metronidazole in prolonged abx-associated diarrhea
- *Aeromonas* - role of therapy unclear, but treat when sx severe; effective abx: cipro, chloramphenicol, TCN, TMP-SMX
- *Plesiomonas* - role of therapy unclear but treat when sx severe; effective abx: cipro, chloramphenicol, TCN, TMP-SMX
- **Tropical sprue** - folate 5 mg/day + vit B_{12} 1000 µg/week + TCN 250 mg qid × 6 months
- *Tropheryma whippelii (Whipple's disease)*:
    1. TMP-SMX bid × 1 year; if sulfa allergic, PCN
    2. supplemental folate, Fe, B_{12}, fat-soluble vitamins

3. periodic re-evaluation due to not infrequent relapse especially in CNS (check CSF)
4. if CNS relapse, repeat 1-year course of TMP-SMX; if unresponsive, chloramphenicol; if non-CNS relapse, TMP-SMX × 1 year; if unresponsive, PCN

Viruses
- ▶ **Rotavirus** - hydration and electrolyte replacement
- ▶ **Norwalk agent** - hydration and electrolyte replacement
- ▶ **CMV** - therapy not indicated in self-limited dz
- ▶ **HSV** – acyclovir

Parasites
- ▶ *Giardia lamblia* - Options:
    1. quinacrine 100 mg tid × 7 days
    2. metronidazole 250 mg tid × 7 days
    3. combination of both
- ▶ *Cryptosporidia* - no effective therapy
- ▶ *Microsporidia* - albendazole 400 mg bid-tid up to 3 months
- ▶ *Isospora belli*
    1. TMP-SMX qid × 7 days then bid × 3 weeks
    2. sulfadiazine 4 g and pyrimethamine 35–75 mg qid + leucovorin calcium 15–25 mg q day × 3–7 weeks
- ▶ *Cyclospora cayetanensis* - TMP-SMX shortens duration of sx
- ▶ *Entamoeba histolytica* - metronidazole 750 mg tid × 10 days with or followed by iodoquinol 650 mg tid × 20 days
- ▶ *Entamoeba coli* - nonpathogenic
- ▶ *Entamoeba hartmanni* - nonpathogenic
- ▶ *Endolimax nana* - nonpathogenic
- ▶ *Iodamoeba buetschlii* - nonpathogenic
- ▶ *Blastocystis hominis* - metronidazole, also responds to TMP-SMX
- ▶ *Balantidium coli* - TCN

TABLE 1-8
INDICATIONS FOR EMPIRIC AND SPECIFIC ANTIMICROBIAL THERAPY IN INFECTIOUS DIARRHEA[a]

Indication	Suggested therapy
Fever (oral temperature >38.5°C) with one of the following: dysentery or those with leukocyte-, lactoferrin-, or hemoccult-positive stools	Quinolone[b]: NF 400 mg, CF 500 mg, OF 300 mg twice a day for 3–5 days
Shigellosis	TMP-SMZ 160 mg/800 mg twice a day for 3 days or quinolone as above
Non-*typhi* species of *Salmonella*	Not routinely recommended, but if severe disease associated with fever and systemic toxicity or important underlying condition use TMP-SMZ 160 mg/800 mg or fluoroquinolone as above for 5–7 days
Campylobacter species	Erythromycin 500 mg twice a day for 5 days
E. coli species	
Enterotoxigenic (ETEC)	TMP-SMZ 160 mg/800 mg twice a day for 3 days or fluoroquinolone twice a day for 3 days
Enteropathogenic (EPEC)	
Enteroadherent (EAEC)	
Enterohemorrhagic (EHEC)	Avoid antimotility agents; role of antibiotics is unclear and they should be avoided
Aeromonas/Plesiomonas	TMP-SMZ 160 mg/800 mg twice a day for 3 days
Vibrio cholerae	Tetracycline 500 mg four times a day for 3 days or doxycycline 300 mg as a single dose
Yersinia species	Antibiotics not usually required; for severe infections use combination therapy with aminoglycoside, doxycycline, TMP-SMZ, or quinolone
Parasites	
Giardia	Metronidazole 250 mg three times a day for 7 days
Cryptosporidium species	None; for severe cases consider paromomycin 500 mg three times a day for 7 days
Cyclospora species	TMP-SMZ 160 mg/800 mg twice a day for 7 days
Entamoeba histolytica	Metronidazole 750 mg three times a day for 10 days plus iodoquinol 650 mg three times a day for 20 days

[a]Adapted from DuPont HL. Guidelines on acute infectious diarrhea in adults. The Practice Parameters Committee of the American College of Gastroenterology. *Am J Gastroenterol* 1997;92:1962.
[b]Fluoroquinolones include norfloxacin (NF), ciprofloxacin (CF), and ofloxacin (OF).

REFERENCES

1. Pardi DS. Microscopic colitis. *Mayo Clin Proc* 2003;78:614–617.
2. Hurley BW, Nguyen CC. The spectrum of pseudomembranous entero-colitis and antibiotic-associated diarrhea. *Arch Intern Med* 2002; 162:2177–2184.
3. Banerjee S, LaMont JT. Treatment of gastrointestinal infections. *Gastroenterology* 2000;118:S48–S67.
4. Fass R, Longstreth GF, Pimental M, et al. Evidence- and consensus-based practice guidelines for the diagnosis of irritable bowel syndrome. *Arch Intern Med* 2001;161:2081–2088.
5. Horwitz BJ, Fisher RS. Irritable bowel syndrome. *N Engl J Med* 2001;344(24):1846–1850.
6. Yassin SF, Young-Fadok TM, Zein NN, et al. Clostridium difficile-associated diarrhea and colitis. *Mayo Clin Proc* 2001;76:725–730.
7. Yamada T, ed. *Handbook of Gastroenterology.* Philadelphia: Lippincott Williams & Wilkins, 1998.
8. McNally PR. *Liver Secrets.* 2nd ed. Philadelphia: Hanley & Belfus, Inc, 2001.
9. Edwards ZC. Gastroenterology. In: Edwards TI, Mayer T, eds. *Urgent Care Medicine.* New York: McGraw-Hill, 2002:327.
10. Abdrabbo K, Peura DA. Update on travelers' diarrhea: practical strategies for prevention and treatment. *Pract Gastroenterol* 2003;XXVII(7):13–24.
11. Seidner DL. Short bowel syndrome: etiology, pathophysiology, and management. *Pract Gastroenterol* 2001;XXV(9):63–72.
12. Abdrabbo K, Peura DA. Giardiasis: a review. *Pract Gastroenterol* 2002;XXVI(6):15–29.
13. Scott BA, Prindiville TP. Microscopic colitis: collagenous colitis and lymphocytic colitis. *Pract Gastroenterol* 2002;XXVI(9):41–51.
14. Mann NS. Management of diabetic diarrhea. *Gastroenterol Endoscop News* 2001;52(7):7–13.

CHAPTER 2

MOTILITY DISORDER SYNDROMES

MOTILITY SYNDROMES
Highlights

► **Helpful in differentiating syndromes:**
  - motility study: esophageal pressure readings, pattern of contractions, pattern of peristalsis
  - symptoms
► **Major Syndromes:**
  - achalasia: occurs as a result of postganglionic denervation of smooth muscle
  - secondary achalasia:
    1. Chagas disease - secondary to *Trypanosoma cruzi* → megaesophagus, megaduodenum, megacolon, megaureter, cardiomyopathy
    2. underlying neoplasm
  - vigorous achalasia
  - diffuse esophageal spasm
  - nutcracker esophagus
  - hypertensive lower esophageal sphincter (LES)
  - nonspecific esophageal motor disorder
  - scleroderma
  - idiopathic intestinal pseudo-obstruction
  - dysphagia with progression from solids to solids and liquids: more common with mechanical obstruction
  - dysphagia to solids and liquids from onset: more common with motor disorders
  - dysphagia related to temperature of food: more common with motor disorders

Required Motility Study Criteria

▶ **Achalasia** - incomplete deglutitive LES relaxation; aperistalsis in smooth muscle esophagus

▶ **Vigorous achalasia** - incomplete deglutitive LES relaxation; simultaneous deglutitive contractions in smooth muscle esophagus (> 40 mm Hg)

▶ **Diffuse esophageal spasm** - simultaneous contractions in smooth muscle with ≥ 30% of swallows

▶ **Nutcracker esophagus** - mean distal esophageal peristaltic amplitude > 180 mm Hg; normal deglutitive LES relaxation; normal peristalsis

▶ **Hypertensive LES** - increased resting LESP (> 40–45 mm Hg); normal deglutitive LES relaxation; normal esoph body peristalsis

▶ **Nonspecific esophageal motor disorder** - peristaltic abnormalities of insufficient severity to establish any of the above diagnoses, yet not thought to be normal

▶ **Scleroderma** - incompetent LES; low-amplitude contractions in smooth muscle of esoph with progression to aperistalsis

Associated Motility Study Findings

Symptoms/Signs/Labs

▶ **Achalasia** - elevated LESP; elevated intra-esoph pressure; dysphagia most prevalent sx (> 90%), regurgitation (> 70%, more common as an early sx), CP (30–50%), weight loss (60%, usually early in course), heartburn, aspiration pneumonia, regurgitant on pillow; x-ray: dilated intrathoracic esoph with air-fluid level, absence of gastric air shadow in AP view, widened mediastinum, "bird's beak," sigmoid esophagus; endoscopy: scope pops through with only gentle pressure, dilated esoph; radionuclide studies: delayed esoph emptying; increased risk of esophageal ca

▶ **Vigorous achalasia** - incomplete deglutitive LES relaxation; simultaneous deglutitive contractions in smooth muscle esophagus (> 40 mm Hg)

▶ **Diffuse esophageal spasm** - repetitive contractions (> 2 peaks); prolonged contractions (> 6 seconds); high amplitude contractions (> 180 mm Hg); spontaneous contractions; corkscrew esophagus on barium; CP most common sx, nonprogressive dysphagia - solids and liquids, cold > hot, weight loss related to sitophobia; regurg rare

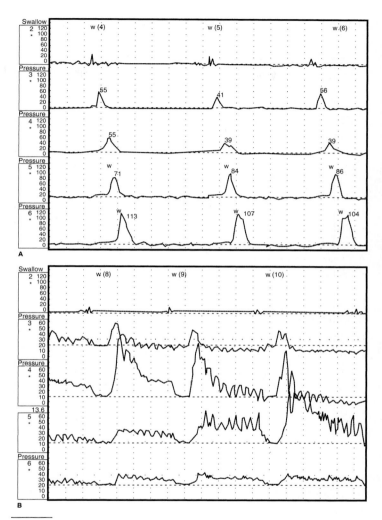

FIGURE 2-1

Normal esophageal motility study. (Reproduced with permission from Friedman SL, McQuaid KR, Grendell JH. *Current Diagnosis & Treatment in Gastroenterology.* Lange Medical Books/McGraw-Hill, 2003.)

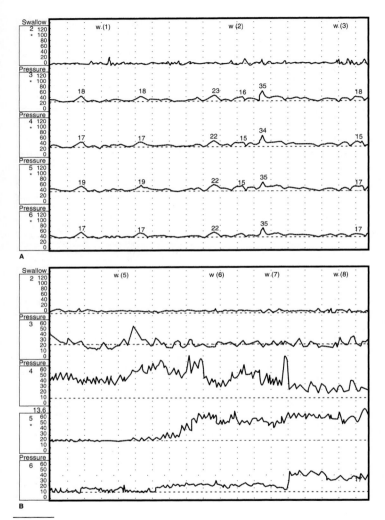

FIGURE 2-2

Esophageal motility study in achalasia. (Reproduced with permission from Friedman SL, McQuaid KR, Grendell JH. *Current Diagnosis & Treatment in Gastroenterology.* Lange Medical Books/McGraw-Hill, 2003.)

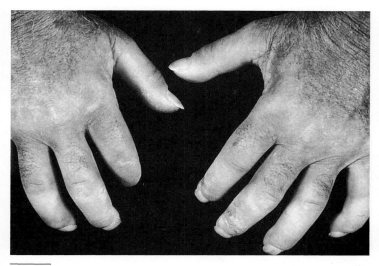

FIGURE 2-3
Scleroderma showing acral sclerosis and focal digital ulcers. (Reproduced with permission from Braunwald E, Fauci AS, Kasper DL, et al. *Harrison's Principles of Internal Medicine.* 16th ed. McGraw-Hill, 2005.)

▶ **Nutcracker esophagus** - repetitive contractions (> 2 peaks); prolonged contractions (> 6 seconds); increased resting LESP (> 40 mm Hg); noncardiac CP

▶ **Hypertensive LES** - incomplete LES relaxation (residual pressure > 8 mm Hg)

▶ **Nonspecific esophageal motor disorder** - frequent nontransmitted contractions (> 20% of swallows); retrograde contractions; repetitive contractions (> 2 peaks); low amplitude contractions (< 30 mm Hg); prolonged contractions (> 6 seconds); high amplitude contractions (> 180 mm Hg); spontaneous contractions; incomplete LES relaxation

▶ **Scleroderma** - heartburn (30–50%), dysphagia, potential stricture from reflux disease (3× more likely than in patients with routine reflux), potential odynophagia/dysphagia related to *Candida*; + ANA in 95%, anti-Scl-70 antigen in 20%, anti-centromere Ab in 50%, anti-nucleolar antibody in 50%

▶ **Idiopathic colonic pseudo-obstruction** - esoph complaints usually only minor

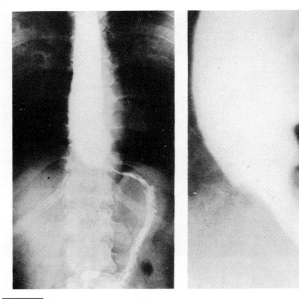

FIGURE 2-4
Achalasia of the esophagus. (Reproduced with permission from Way LW, Doherty GM. *Current Surgical Diagnosis & Treatment.* Lange Medical Books/McGraw-Hill, 2003.)

Treatment

► **Achalasia** - Botox injection (30–50% response rate); pneumatic dilation (70% response rate); surgery - Heller myotomy + fundoplication prn (90% response rate)
► **Vigorous achalasia** - variable response to smooth muscle relaxants
► **Diffuse esophageal spasm (DES)** - No therapeutic agents have demonstrated efficacy for DES.
► **Nutcracker esophagus** - can try NTG, calcium channel blockers: nifedipine, diltiazem
► **Hypertensive LES** - variable response to smooth muscle relaxants
► **Nonspecific esophageal motor disorder** - No therapeutic agents have demonstrated efficacy for any of the nonspecific disorders in controlled trials.
► **Scleroderma** - treatment of reflux disease

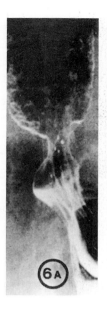

FIGURE 2-5
Esophagram of scleroderma. (Reproduced with permission from Braunwald E, Fauci AS, Kasper DL, et al. *Harrison's Principles of Internal Medicine.* 16th ed. McGraw-Hill, 2005.)

Miscellaneous: Small Bowel and Colonic Motility

► myopathy → hypoactive musculature
► neuropathy → hyperactive musculature
► IAS (internal anal sphincter) - smooth muscle
► EAS (external anal sphincter) - striated muscle
  • types of incontinence:
    1. reservoir
    2. overflow
    3. rectosphincteric
► IBS tx - 5HT3 antagonist for diarrhea, 5HT4 agonist for constipation
► disorders of defecation:
  • weak propulsion → megarectum, pain syndromes
  • misdirection of propulsion → rectocele
  • failure of IAS relaxation → Hirschsprung's disease

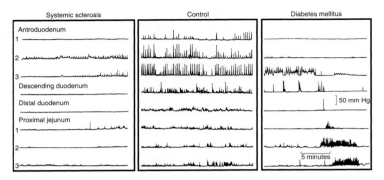

FIGURE 2-6
Small bowel motility study in myopathy and neuropathy. (Reproduced with permission from Friedman SL, McQuaid KR, Grendell JH. *Current Diagnosis & Treatment in Gastroenterology.* Lange Medical Books/McGraw-Hill, 2003.)

- • failure of puborectalis muscle (PRM) and EAS relaxation → pelvic floor dyssynergia
- ▶ indications for surgery (subtotal colectomy with ileorectal anastomosis) in intractable constipation:
  - • chronic, severe, disabling sx
  - • unresponsive to medical tx
  - • no intestinal dysmotility
  - • normal anorectal function
- ▶ excitatory small bowel neurotransmitters - substance P, serotonin
- ▶ inhibitory small bowel neurotransmitters - nitric oxide, VIP
- ▶ enteric myopathy - contractions of low amplitude, MMCs peristaltic but of low amplitude
- ▶ enteric neuropathy - extrinsic denervation (vagus and sympathetic), intrinsic denervation (enteric nervous system), fasting motility pattern normal, impaired response to meal; ↓ postprandial and contractile activity
- ▶ intrinsic neuropathy - contractions of normal amplitude, fasting ↓ MMC, abnormal propagation of MMC and clustered contractions
- ▶ fed - absent or incomplete conversion to fed pattern, premature return to fasting pattern
- ▶ localized bowel obstruction - repeated clusters of contraction in normal proximal bowel

▶ Hirschsprung's disease - congenital disorder (autosomal dominant: RET gene; autosomal recessive: endothelin-B receptor gene)
  • male:female = 5:1
  • obstipation/constipation from birth, colonic dilatation proximal to spastic nonpropulsive segment of distal small bowel
  • aganglionosis of submucosal and myenteric plexuses
  • bx: + acetylcholinesterase stain
  • barium study: spastic, nonpropulsive, segment of distal bowel with colonic dilation proximally
  • anal manometry: absence of IAS relaxation after rectal distension
  • tx:
    1. short and ultrashort segment - anal myotomy
    2. long segment - may need to consider bypass or resection of denervated segment
▶ colonic inertia - slow colonic transit of proximal colon, normal colon diameter, ↓ high amplitude peristaltic contractions, ↓ response to meals/cholinergics/laxatives, delayed passage of markers through proximal colon
▶ outlet delay - slow rectosigmoid colon transit, + megarectum
▶ pelvic floor dyssynergia - need ≥ 2 studies positive: anorectal manometry, anal sphincter EMG, defecography, impaired balloon expulsion from rectum, failure of relaxation of the PRM during attempted defecation

REFERENCES

1. Hirano I. Achalasia. *Clin Perspect Gastroenterol* 2002;5(3):165–172.
2. Firth M, Prather CM. Gastrointestinal motility problems in the elderly patient. *Gastroenterology* 2002;122:1688–1700.
3. Pandolfino JE, Howden CW, Kahrilas PJ. Motility-modifying agents and management of disorders of gastrointestinal motility. *Gastroenterology* 2000;118:S32–S47.
4. Wong RKH, guest ed. Achalasia. In: *Gastrointestinal Endoscopy Clinics of North America*. Philadelphia: W.B. Saunders, 2001.
5. Yamada Y, ed. *Textbook of Gastroenterology*. 3rd ed. Philadelphia: Lippincott Williams & Wilkins, 1999.
6. Goldman L, Bennett JC, eds. *Cecil Textbook of Medicine*. 21st ed. Philadelphia: W.B. Saunders, 2000.

CHAPTER 3

INTESTINAL ISCHEMIA SYNDROMES

INTESTINAL ISCHEMIA SYNDROMES
Highlights

► **Helpful in differentiating syndromes:**
  • site of disease in GI tract
  • symptoms and demographics
  • findings on radiologic imaging and endoscopic studies

► **Major Syndromes:**
  • acute mesenteric ischemia - arterial (AMI):
    1. superior mesenteric artery emboli (SAME)
    2. non-occlusive mesenteric ischemia (NOMI)
    3. superior mesenteric artery thrombosis (SMAT)
  • mesenteric venous thrombosis (MVI)
    1. acute
    2. chronic
  • focal segmental ischemia (FSI)
  • chronic mesenteric ischemia (CMI) (aka intestinal angina)
  • colonic ischemia (CI)

► colon ischemia (CI) twice as common as acute mesenteric ischemic (AMI) syndromes

► AMI involves GI tract supplied by SMA and its branches

► arterial causes > venous causes of AMI

► embolic disease > thrombotic disease in AMI

► AMI - usually present during ischemic episode

► CI - usually present after ischemic episode

► angiography with infusion of vasodilators integral part of diagnosis and management of AMI

▶ AMI accounts for only 33% of all episodes of intestinal ischemia but aids majority of ischemia-related mortality

▶ SMA emboli (SAME) 50%, non-occlusive mesenteric ischemia (NOMI) 30%, SMA thrombosis (SMAT) 10%

Demographics

▶ **Acute mesenteric ischemia - arterial (AMI):**

  • *superior mesenteric artery emboli (SAME):* emboli usually from L atrial or ventricular mural thrombus; many patients with h/o of previous peripheral emboli and 20% with synchronous emboli to other arteries

  • *non-occlusive mesenteric ischemia (NOMI):* results from splanchnic vasoconstriction from preceding cardiovascular event; ↑ risk with hemodialysis or major cardiac or intra-abdominal surgery; pain absent in 25%

  • *superior mesenteric artery thrombosis (SMAT):* occurs at areas of severe atherosclerotic narrowing, most often at origin of SMA; commonly superimposed on CI, with 20–50% with h/o intestinal angina; frequent h/o coronary, cerebral, or peripheral arterial ischemia

▶ **Mesenteric venous thrombosis (MVT):** seen in 5–10% of AMI cases; etiology: BCP, antithrombin III, protein S and C deficiency, polycythemia vera, myeloproliferative disorder; 20–50% mortality

▶ **Focal segmental ischemia (FSI)** - etiology: atheromatous emboli, strangulated hernia, vasculitis, blunt abdominal trauma, XRT; usually adequate collateral circulation to avoid infarction

▶ **Chronic mesenteric ischemia (CMI)** (aka intestinal angina) - < 5% of cases of intestinal ischemia; almost always caused by mesenteric atherosclerosis

▶ **Colonic ischemia (CI)** - most common ischemic disorder of GI tract; etiology: vasculitis especially SLE, sickle cell, coagulopathy, cocaine, long distance running, Rx - estrogen, NSAIDs; idiopathic in most cases; splenic flexure, descending colon, and sigmoid most common sites; complication of aortic surgery in 1–7% of cases, as high as 60% of cases of aortic rupture, and responsible for 10% of deaths in aortic surgery; obstructive lesion in 10–15% of cases: colon ca, stricture, diverticulitis, volvulus, fecal impaction, XRT stricture

TABLE 3-1
PATTERNS OF INTESTINAL ISCHEMIA

Condition	Etiology	Clinical features	Management
Mesenteric artery embolus	Arterial embolus associated with atrial fibrillation or rheumatic heart disease	Acute central abdominal pain, shock, peritonitis	Immediate angiography and embolectomy if possible
Abdominal angina	Atherosclerosis of celiac and superior mesenteric arteries	Chronic postprandial pain, weight loss	Angiography and surgery in selected cases
Ischemic colitis	Low-flow state	Acute lower abdominal pain, rectal bleeding	Sigmoidoscopy; surgery only for peritonitis

Symptoms/Signs/Labs

▶ **Acute mesenteric ischemia - arterial (AMI):** acute abdominal pain out of proportion to physical findings; 75% with WBC > 15K, 50% with metabolic acidemia; "thumb-printing" on plain films of small bowel or R colon and ⇒ intestinal infarction
  • *superior mesenteric artery emboli (SAME)*
  • *non-occlusive mesenteric ischemia (NOMI)*
  • *superior mesenteric artery thrombosis (SMAT)*
▶ **Mesenteric venous thrombosis (MVT):**
  • *acute:* abdominal pain initially out of proportion to physical findings, N&V and occult blood in 50%; gross GIB in 15% and ⇒ infarction, fever; duration of sx 1–2 weeks before admission
  • *chronic:* asymptomatic or GI bleeding usually from esophageal varices; physical findings of portal hypertension
▶ **Focal segmental ischemia (FSI):**
  • 3 presentations:
    1. acute enteritis - simulates appendicitis
    2. chronic enteritis - may simulate Crohn's disease
    3. obstruction - most common
  • may see "sentinel loop" or tapered stricture on imaging
▶ **Chronic mesenteric ischemia (CMI)** (aka intestinal angina) - cardinal feature: meal-associated abdominal pain within 30 minutes with increasing severity and then gradual abatement

over 1–3 hours; expect to see food aversion and weight loss; abdominal bruit common

▶ **Colonic ischemia (CI):**
- presentations:
  1. reversible colopathy (~ 2/3)
  2. transient colitis (~ 1/3)
  3. perforation and gangrene
  4. stricture
  5. chronic segmental colitis
  6. fulminant colitis
- sx: mild, LLQ pain, urge to defecate, bright red or maroon blood mixed with stool
- may be confused with IBD or infectious colitis
- sx resolution usually 24–48 hours and healing usually within 2 weeks

Diagnosis

▶ **Acute mesenteric ischemia - arterial (AMI):**
- *superior mesenteric artery emboli (SAME)*
- *non-occlusive mesenteric ischemia (NOMI)*
- *superior mesenteric artery thrombosis (SMAT)*
  1. selective mesenteric angiography mainstay
  2. CT to rule out other causes of sx
▶ **Mesenteric venous thrombosis (MVT):**
- *acute:*
  1. CT scan diagnostic in 90%:
     - thickening and enhancement of bowel wall
     - enlarged SMV with central lucency
     - dilated collateral vessels
  2. selective mesenteric angiography
▶ **Chronic mesenteric ischemia (CMI)** (aka intestinal angina):
  1. Doppler U/S, MRA, or spiral CT for screening
  2. if screening test(s) abnormal, follow with splanchnic angiography - usually see at least 2 of 3 splanchnic vessels either completely obstructed or severely stenosed
▶ **Colonic ischemia (CI)** - colonoscopy within 48 hours of sx - hemorrhagic nodules with F/U
▶ exam 1 week later which may show normal colon, evolution with segmental ulceration

Treatment

▶ **Acute mesenteric ischemia - arterial (AMI):**
- *superior mesenteric artery emboli (SAME)*
- *non-occlusive mesenteric ischemia (NOMI)*
- *superior mesenteric artery thrombosis (SMAT)*
  1. treat precipitating cause
  2. Papaverine should not be used in patients in shock.
  3. thrombolytic therapy if:
     - partially occluding embolus
     - embolus in branch of SMA or main SMA distal to ileocolic artery
       and
     - study performed within 24° of sx
  4. laparotomy prn, including second look 12–24 hours later

▶ **Mesenteric venous thrombosis (MVT):**
- *acute:*
  1. trial of heparin or thrombolytic therapy if no evidence of infarction
  2. laparotomy if infarction present + heparinization × 7–10 days followed by Coumadin × 3 months
- *chronic:* focused on treatment of sequelae of portal hypertension; if asxtic, treatment usually not necessary

▶ **Focal segmental ischemia (FSI)** - resection of involved bowel

▶ **Chronic mesenteric ischemia (CMI)** (aka intestinal angina) - revascularization procedure: surgery vs. angioplasty

▶ **Colonic ischemia (CI):**
  1. expectant:
     - IVF
     - abx
     - optimization of cardiac function
     - serial evaluation
  2. laparotomy for infarction

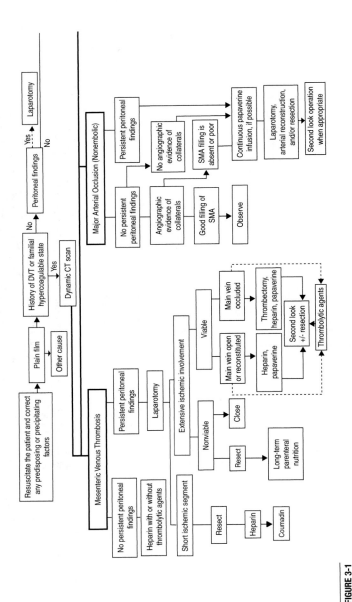

FIGURE 3-1

Algorithm for diagnosis and treatment of acute intestinal ischemia. (Reproduced with permission from Friedman SL, McQuaid KR, Grendell JH. Current Diagnosis & Treatment in Gastroenterology. Lange Medical Books/McGraw-Hill, 2003.)

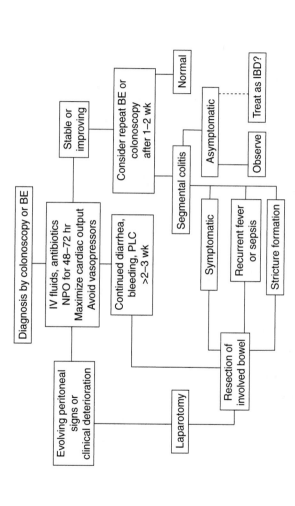

FIGURE 3-2

Management of colon ischemia. (Reproduced with permission from Friedman SL, McQuaid KR, Grendell JH. Current Diagnosis & Treatment in Gastroenterology. Lange Medical Books/McGraw-Hill, 2003.)

REFERENCES

1. Yamada T, ed. *Handbook of Gastroenterology*. Philadelphia: Lippincott Williams & Wilkins, 1998.
2. McNally P. *GI/Liver Secrets*. 2nd ed. Philadelphia: Hanley & Belfus Inc, 2001.
3. Feldman M, Scharschmidt BF, Sleisenger MH. *Sleisenger & Fordtran's Gastrointestinal and Liver Disease*. 6th ed. Philadelphia: W.B. Saunders Co, 1998.
4. Yamada Y, ed. *Textbook of Gastroenterology*. 3rd ed. Philadelphia: Lippincott Williams & Wilkins, 1999.
5. Friedman SL, McQuaid KR, Grendell JH. *Diagnosis & Treatment in Gastroenterology*. New York: Lange Medical Books/McGraw-Hill, 2003.

CHAPTER 4

POLYPOSIS AND COLON CANCER SYNDROMES

POLYPOSIS AND COLON CANCER SYNDROMES
Highlights

► **Helpful in differentiating syndromes:**
   - genetic profile
   - symptoms, demographics, presence/absence of extraintestinal manifestations
   - location and morphology of polyps
► **Major Syndromes:**
   - familial adenomatous polyposis (FAP):
     - Gardner's syndrome
     - Crails syndrome
     - Turcot's syndrome
     - AFAP (attenuated FAP)
   - I1307K APC gene mutation
   - Peutz-Jeghers syndrome
   - solitary juvenile polyposis syndrome
   - juvenile polyposis coli
   - Bannayan-Ruvalcaba-Riley syndrome (Bannayan-Zonana)
   - Gorlin syndrome
   - Cowden's syndrome
   - Basal Cell Nevus syndrome
   - Cronkhite-Canada syndrome
   - hyperplastic polyposis
   - Lynch syndrome (hereditary nonpolyposis colon ca):
     - Lynch I: multiple primary cancers restricted to colon and no family history of other cancers

- Lynch II (cancer family syndrome) associated with ↑ familial occurrence of other forms of cancer, especially breast, uterine, and ovarian
- Muir-Torré syndrome

Demographics

► **Familial adenomatous polyposis (FAP)** - autosomal dominant; mutation of APC gene on chromosome 5q21; 1 in 8300–1:14,000 births; 2nd leading cause of death is ca of 2nd portion of duodenum (5–10%), 100% risk of colon ca
  - Gardner's syndrome: if extraintestinal manifestations present in FAP
  - Crails syndrome: FAP variant with medulloblastoma of brain
  - Turcot's syndrome: MMR mutation, oligopolyposis, malignant CNS tumors (glioblastoma, medulloblastoma, astrocytoma, ependymoma); can be seen as variant of hereditary nonpolyposis colon ca (HNPCC); mutation of mismatch repair gene
  - AFAP (attenuated FAP): 6% of FAP pedigrees, 100% risk of colon ca but 10–15 years later than FAP, oligopolyposis, plethora of upper tract lesions (fundic gland polyps, duodenal adenomas, periampullary ca)
► **1307K APC gene mutation** - autosomal dominant, seen in Ashkenazi Jews, 1.4–1.9-fold increased risk of colon ca; 6% carrier frequency
► **Peutz-Jeghers syndrome** - autosomal dominant, mutation of STK11 gene on chromosome 19p, 93% develop at least one ca, with 54% of females developing breast ca
► **Solitary juvenile polyposis syndrome** - non-inherited, no increased risk of ca
► **Juvenile polyposis coli** - autosomal dominant, 21% with DPC4 (also called SMAD4) on chromosome 18q21, mutation in PTEN gene; 20–70% risk of colon ca, increased risk of gastric, small bowel, and pancreatic ca as well as arteriovenous and cardiovascular malformations
► **Bannayan-Ruvalcaba-Riley syndrome (Bannayan-Zonana)** - possibly autosomal dominant, ? variant of juvenile polyposis, mutation in PTEN gene on chromosome 10q in 50–60%
► **Gorlin syndrome** - mutation of TCH gene on chromosome 9q
► **Cowden's syndrome** - autosomal dominant, mutation of PTEN gene on chromosome 10q in 80%

▶ **Basal Cell Nevus syndrome** - gastric hamartomatous polyps, basal cell ca

▶ **Cronkhite-Canada syndrome** - nonfamilial, most cases seen in Japan

▶ **Hyperplastic polyposis** - autosomal dominant, high risk of colon ca

▶ **Lynch syndrome (HNPCC)** - autosomal dominant, accounts for 3% of colon ca cases, HNPCC gene mutation - hMSH2 on chromosome 2p16 and hMLH1 on chromosome 3p21 account for 95% of gene changes seen, 70–80% risk of colon ca and occurs at younger age (avg of 44), increased risk of extracolonic ca; rule of **1-2-3: 1** relative < 50 yo with colon ca; ≥ **2** generations affected; **3** affected relatives, one of whom is 1st degree relative of the other two

  • Lynch I: multiple primary cancers restricted to colon and no family history of other cancers
  • Lynch II (cancer family syndrome): associated with ↑ familial occurrence of other forms of cancer, especially breast, uterine, and ovarian

▶ **Muir-Torré syndrome** - variant of HNPCC

Symptoms/Signs/Labs

▶ **Familial adenomatous polyposis (FAP)** - ≥100 adenomas throughout colon; extracolonic/extraintestinal manifestations:
  • *markers: radiopaque jaw lesions, microadenomas, *CHRPE* (congenital hypertrophy of retinal pigment epithelium) lesions; ≥3 CHRPE lesions - 100% predictive value
  • extracolonic polyps: small bowel, stomach (including fundic gland retention polyps in 50–90%)
  • cutaneous lesions: lipoma, fibroma, sebaceous and *epidermoid* cysts
  • other: *CHRPE*, *desmoid tumor*, *periampullary ca*, *osteoma*, dental abnormalities, nasopharyngeal angiofibroma - *extracolonic ca: periampullary ca*, hepatoblastoma, thyroid, duodenal, pancreas, brain, biliary tree; angiofibroma of nares in teenage males

▶ **Turcot's syndrome** - adenomatous oligopolyposis + brain tumors (glioblastoma and astrocytoma)

▶ **Peutz-Jeghers syndrome** - *hamartomatous polyps* (arborization of smooth muscle on path) in small bowel but also seen in colon

TABLE 4-1
GENES ALTERED IN SPORADIC COLORECTAL CANCER

Gene	Chromosome	Tumors with alterations (%)	Class	Function
K-ras	12	50	Proto-oncogene	Encodes guanine nucleotide-binding protein that regulates intracellular signaling
APC	5	70	Tumor suppressor	Regulation of β-catenin involved in activation of Wnt/TcF signaling (activates c-myc, cyclin D1),[a] regulation of proliferation, apoptosis; interaction with E-cadherin (? cell adhesion)
DCC	18	70	? Tumor suppressor	Neutrin-1 receptor; caspase substrate in apoptosis; cell adhesion
SMAD4 (DPC4, MADH4)	18	?	Tumor suppressor	Nuclear transcription factor in TGF-β1 signaling; regulation of angiogenesis; regulator of WAF1 promoter; downstream mediator of SMAD2
p53	17	75	Tumor suppressor	Transcription factor; regulator of cell cycle progression after cellular stress, of apoptosis, of gene expression, and of DNA repair
hMSH2	2	—[b]	DNA mismatch repair	Maintains fidelity of DNA replication
hMLH1	3	—[b]	DNA mismatch repair	Maintains fidelity of DNA replication
hMSH6	2	—[c]	DNA mismatch repair	Maintains fidelity of DNA replication
TGF-β1 RII	3	—[c]	Tumor suppressor	Receptor for signaling in the TGF-β1 pathway; inhibitor of colonic epithelial proliferation, often mutated in tumors with MSI

[a]β-Catenin mutations (downstream of APC) are found in 16–25% of microsatellite instability (MSI) colon cancers, but not in microsatellite stable (MSS) cancers.
[b]Approximately 15% of sporadic colorectal cancers demonstrate MSI associated with alterations in mismatch repair genes (principally hMSH2 and hMLH1 but also hMSH3, hMSH6, hPMS1, and hPMS2).
[c]Mutated in 73–90% of MSI colon cancers. Up to 55% of MSS colon cancer cell lines may demonstrate a TGF-β signaling blockage distal to TGF-β1 RII.

and stomach, *brown macular melanin pigmentation* on lips/buccal mucosa/hands/feet/eye lids which fades at puberty; children: small bowel intussusception; adults: increased risk of ca of *breast*, *colon*, stomach, ovary (Sertoli cell tumor), lung, small bowel, uterus (adenoma malignum of cervix), esophagus, testes; path of polyp: arborization of smooth muscle

▶ **Solitary juvenile polyposis syndrome** - presentation of 1–2 polyps in rectosigmoid at avg age of 4 with rectal bleeding or anal prolapse of polyp

▶ **Juvenile polyposis coli** - ≥5 juvenile hamartomatous polyps, with up to 100's of polyps in colorectum but also seen in small bowel and stomach; usual presentation - anemia, rectal bleeding, failure to thrive, abdominal pain, hypoalbuminemia in late childhood/early adolescence; path of polyp - edematous mucosa with cystic dilation

▶ **Bannayan-Ruvalcaba-Riley syndrome (Bannayan-Zonana)** - juvenile polyps, craniofacial appearance, developmental delay, macrocephaly, pigmented macules on shaft and glans of penis, lipid storage myopathy

▶ **Gorlin syndrome** - multiple nevoid basal carcinomas, skeletal abnormalities, odontogenic keratinocytes, macrocephaly, intracranial calcification, craniofacial abnormalities

▶ **Cowden's syndrome** - cardinal feature: *multiple facial trichilemmomas* (orocutaneous hamartomas) in > 90%, occurring around mouth, nose, eyes, variable hamartomatous involvement of GI tract (35%), skin, mucous membranes, thyroid, breast, adnexa; verrucous skin lesions of face and limbs, cobblestone-like papules of gingiva, buccal mucosa, and tongue; extraintestinal lesions - adenomas and cysts of thyroid (70%), *thyroid ca* (3%), fibrocystic dz and *fibroadenomas of breast* (52%), *breast ca* (28%), *GYN ca* in 60%

▶ **Cronkhite-Canada syndrome** - multiple juvenile polyps in GI tract (except esoph), cutaneous hyperpigmentation, hair loss, nail dystrophy, protein-losing enteropathy; presenting sx - diarrhea from *protein-losing enteropathy*, weight loss, peripheral edema, fat and disaccharide malabsorption; path - mucosa between polyps with edema, congestion, and inflammation of lamina propria and focal glandular ectasia

▶ **Hyperplastic polyposis** - 100's of hyperplastic polyps
▶ **Lynch syndrome (hereditary nonpolyposis colon ca)** - oligo-polyposis, with polyps predominantly in proximal or R colon; phenotypic signs - café au lait spots, sebaceous glans tumors, keratoacanthomas, extracolonic cancers - *endometrial* (39%), *ovarian* (9%), transitional cell ca of ureter and renal pelvis, adenocarcinoma of stomach, small bowel, ovary, and biliary system
- Lynch I: multiple primary cancers restricted to colon and no family history of other cancers
- Lynch II (cancer family syndrome): associated with ↑ familial occurrence of other forms of cancer, esp breast, uterine, and ovarian
▶ **Muir-Torré syndrome** - oligopolyposis + skin lesions: characterized by either a sebaceous adenoma, sebaceous epithelioma, or sebaceous ca + colon ca in 47%, also basal cell and squamous cell skin ca

Screening

▶ **Familial adenomatous polyposis (FAP)**
- begin testing for APC gene at age 10–12
- if gene testing not done, yearly flex starting at age 12
- after age 50, AGA guidelines for avg-risk patient
- consider screening for hepatoblastoma from age 0–5
▶ **1307K APC gene mutation** - gene testing
▶ **Peutz-Jeghers syndrome**
- STK11 gene testing
- screening in 1st degree relatives at least once early in 2nd decade of life with UGI w/SBFT
- affected patients - upper and lower endo w/ bx and polypectomy and small bowel x-ray q 2 years
- annual H&P + labs + baseline mammogram at age 25, then yearly; at age 40 + yearly pelvic and pelvic U/S beginning in adolescence + CA-125 starting at age 18 + breast and testicular self-exam
▶ **Juvenile polyposis coli:**
- initial screening of 1st degree relatives with colonoscopy at age 12
- subsequent screening with flex + hemoccult q 3–5 years

- gene testing not commercially available
- complete upper and lower endo + small bowel imaging with bx of flat mucosa and polyps q 1–3 years + polypectomy prn

▶ **Cowden's syndrome:**
  - annual H&P with special attention to neck (looking for thyroid dz) starting at age 18 or 5 years earlier than youngest age of diagnosis + breast exam at age 25 with mammogram at age 30 or 5 years earlier than youngest age of diagnosis + endometrial bx at age 35 or 5 years earlier than youngest age of diagnosis + annual urinalysis

▶ **Hyperplastic polyposis** - biopsy to rule out FAP, surveillance for malignant transformation

▶ **Lynch syndrome (hereditary nonpolyposis colon ca):**
  - if gene testing is positive, colonoscopy starting at age 25 or 5 years earlier than youngest age of diagnosis, whichever comes first, and annually thereafter
  - if no genetic testing done, 1st degree relatives to have colonoscopy q 1–2 years starting at age 20–25 and annually after age 40
  - annual screening for endometrial cancer beginning at age 25–35 with endometrial aspiration or transvaginal U/S

Treatment

▶ **Familial adenomatous polyposis (FAP):**
  - colectomy with ileoanal anastomosis at time of diagnosis (if untx'd, avg age of death at 42 due to colon ca)
  - post-op F/U:
    a. q 6 months flex if rectum or pouch remains after surgery
    b. upper endoscopy with side-viewing scope q 6 months–q 4 years
    c. annual exam of thyroid + U/S
    d. sulindac to help prevent polyp formation

▶ **Peutz-Jeghers syndrome** - surgery for sxtic polyps or polyps ≥1.5 cm

▶ **Juvenile polyposis coli** - colectomy (subtotal colectomy with ileoanal anastomosis) when surveillance not possible or persistent bleeding or refractory protein loss

TABLE 4-2
COLORECTAL CANCER SCREENING STRATEGIES FOR PATIENTS AT INCREASED RISK[a]

	Recommendation
Personal History	
History of colon cancer	Evaluate entire colon around the time of resection, then colonoscopy every 3–5 years
History of colonic adenomas	Colonoscopy every 3–5 years
Ulcerative pancolitis of 8 years duration, left-sided colitis >15 years	Colonoscopy with biopsies every 1–3 years
Family History	
Familial adenomatous polyposis	Consider genetic testing
	Annual sigmoidoscopy beginning at age 10–12, consider colectomy when polyps develop; if no polyps, annual sigmoidoscopy until age 40, then every 3–5 years
Hereditary nonpolyposis colorectal cancer (HNPCC)	Consider genetic testing
	Colonoscopy every 2 years beginning at age 25 or when 5 years younger than the youngest affected relative; annual colonoscopy after age 40
Two first-degree relatives with colorectal cancer or adenomas	Colonoscopy every 3–5 years, beginning when 10 years younger than the youngest affected relative
One first-degree relative with sporadic colorectal cancer or adenoma before age 60	Same as above

[a]Adapted from *Screening and Surveillance Colonoscopy in Individuals at Increased Risk for Colorectal Cancer*, American Society for Gastrointestinal Endoscopy, 1998.

▶ **Bannayan-Ruvalcaba-Riley syndrome (Bannayan-Zonana)** - surgery required in most due to too numerous to count (TNTC) polyps
  a. supportive therapy + enteral/parenteral nutrition
  b. steroids if deterioration in condition
  c. surgery for bleeding, ca, intussusception
  d. colonoscopic screening for dysplasia and ca
▶ **Lynch syndrome (hereditary nonpolyposis colon ca)** - subtotal colectomy with ileorectal anastomosis + postsurgical rectal surveillance q 6 months

TABLE 4-3
COLON CANCER

Risk Factor	Cumulative Risk	% of Colon Cancer Cases
• No predisposing risk factors		75%
• Family history of colon ca:		15–20%
– one 1st-degree relative	2–3×	
– two 1st-degree relatives	3–6×	
– 1st-degree relative age < 50	3–6×	
– one 2nd- or 3rd-degree relative	1.5×	
– two 2nd-degree relatives	2–3×	
• Hereditary nonpolyposis colorectal cancer (HNPCC)		4–7%
• Familial adenomatous polyposis (FAP)		1%
• ↑ risk:		
– prior history of endometrial or ovarian cancer		
– saturated fat	2.5×	
– obesity	3× risk (of adenomatous polyps)	
– abdominal obesity	1.8× (of colon cancer) 2.5× (of adenomatous polyps)	
– ETOH and tobacco		
• ↓ risk:		
– exercise	0.5×	
– calcium		
– asa/NSAID (sulindac)/ Cox-2 inhibitor (Celebrex)		
– folate		
– estrogen		

REFERENCES

1. Alley EW, Haller DG. Advances in chemotherapy for colorectal cancer. *Gastroenterol Endosc News* 2002;53(9):31–34.
2. Alley EW, Haller DG. Advances in chemotherapy for colorectal cancer. *Gastroenterol Endosc News* 2001;52(7):31–34.
3. Frank BB. Updates on colorectal cancer screening and prevention. *Gastroenterol Endosc News* 2002;53(7):61–63.
4. Rex DK. Current colorectal cancer screening strategies: overview and obstacles to implementation. *Rev Gastroenterological Dis* 2002;2(suppl 1):S2–S11.

5. Choi SW, Mason JB. Nutritional chemoprevention of colorectal cancer. *Clin Perspect Gastroenterol* 2000;3(5):259–266.

6. Burt RW. Polyposis syndromes. *Clin Perspect Gastroenterol* 2002;5(1):51–59.

7. Ahlquist DA, guest editor. Colorectal cancer prevention and detection. In: *Gastroenterology Clinics of North America* 2002;31(4):926–1181. Philadelphia: W.B. Saunders.

8. Coruz-Correa M, et al. Long-term treatment with sulindac in familial adenomatous polyposis: a prospective cohort study. *Gastroenterology* 2002;122:541–545.

9. Burt RW. Colon cancer screening. *Gastroenterology* 2000;119:837–853.

10. Jarvinen HJ, Aarnio M, Mustonen H, et al. Controlled 15-year trial on screening for colorectal cancer in families with hereditary nonpolyposis colorectal cancer. *Gastroenterology* 2000;118:829–834.

11. Clinical Practice and Practice Economics Committee. American Gastroenterological Association Medical Position Statement: impact of dietary fiber on colon cancer occurrence. *Gastroenterology* 2000;118:1233–1234.

12. Winawer S, Fletcher R, Rex D, et al. Colorectal cancer screening and surveillance: clinical guidelines and rationale—update based on new evidence. *Gastroenterology* 2003;124:544–560.

13. Grady WM. Genetic testing for high-risk colon cancer patients. *Gastroenterology* 2003;124:1574–1594.

14. Imperiale TF, Wagner DR, Lin CY, et al. Results of screening colonoscopy among persons 40 to 49 years of age. *N Engl J Med* 2002;346(23):1781–1785.

15. US Preventive Services Task Force. Screening for colorectal cancer: recommendation and rationale. *Ann Intern Med* 2002;137:129–131.

16. Swaroop VS, Larson MV. Colonoscopy as a screening test for colorectal cancer in average-risk individuals. *Mayo Clin Proc* 2002;77:951–956.

17. Calvert PM, Frucht H. The genetics of colorectal cancer. *Ann Intern Med* 2002;137:603–612.

18. Ransohoff DF, Sandler RS. Screening for colorectal cancer. *N Engl J Med* 2002;346(1):40–44.

19. Chung DC, Rustgi AK. The hereditary nonpolyposis colorectal cancer syndrome: genetics and clinical implications. *Ann Intern Med* 2003;138:560–570.

CHAPTER 5

INFLAMMATORY BOWEL DISEASE

INFLAMMATORY BOWEL DISEASE
General Information

► **Ulcerative colitis** - occurs in both sexes with typical onset in the 2nd through 4th decades of life; confined to the large bowel, though the terminal ileum may be affected (backwash ileitis); diseased segment of bowel is continuous; inflammation occurs in the mucosa and submucosa (the muscularis and serosa are normal); the mucosa may be granular, swollen, friable and may contain pseudopolyps; microscopically the mucosa and submucosa show infiltration with acute and chronic inflammatory cells; the mucosa is atrophic with a diminished quantity of goblet cells and many crypt abscesses; ca risk increases with early onset of dz, total large bowel involvement, dz > 10 years, and chronic inflammation

► **Crohn's colitis** - can occur anywhere in the GI tract from the mouth to the anus; patchy dz with normal bowel present between affected areas; transmural inflammation with submucosal edema, lymphoid aggregation, and fibrosis; submucosal inflammation has a "cobblestone" appearance; the bowel wall becomes thick, rigid, and displays creeping of the fat from the mesentery to the bowel wall in severe or chronic dz; hallmark of dz is sarcoidlike epithelioid granulomas

Symptoms/Signs/Labs

► **Ulcerative colitis** - characterized by exacerbations and remissions; onset may be insidious or abrupt; blood per rectum and diarrhea are the most common symptoms; severe dz may

TABLE 5-1
INFLAMATORY BOWEL DISEASE COMPARATOR

	Ulcerative colitis (UC)	Crohn's disease (CD)
Labs – pANCA positive, ASCA negative	✓ in 75%	
– pANCA negative, ASCA positive		✓ in 86%
Tobacco	• Improvement with use • Exacerbation with cessation • UC more common in nonsmokers & ex-smokers	• worsens with use and dose-related (i.e., # cigs) • CD more common in smokers

Colonic involvement	• 99% with rectal involvement
	• 25% with dz limited to rectum
	• < 20% with pancolitis
		• 45% ileocolonic
		• 33% small bowel only
		• 20% colon only
		• perianal fistulas in 37%
		• distribution:
		  – segmental 40%
		  – total 31%
		  – L colon 26%

Colon cancer	multiple, arises from flat mucosa, infiltrates broadly, uniformly distributed, anaplastic, occurs at younger age than CD	

pANCA, perinuclear anti-neutrophilic cytoplasmic antibodies; ASCA, anti-Saccharomyces cerevisiae.

evoke abd pain and distention, fever, tachycardia, and elevated WBC

▶ **Crohn's disease -** characterized by exacerbations and remissions; onset is insidious; symptoms include nonbloody diarrhea, abd pain, weight loss, anemia, and hypoproteinemia

▶ **Toxic megacolon -** life-threatening complication of both ulcerative colitis (UC) and Crohn's disease; can occur during an acute exacerbation of chronic dz, but usually occurs during the initial presentation; acute colitis with segmental or total dilatation of the colon and accompanying fever, abd pain and tenderness, tachycardia, and leukocytosis; treat with antibiotics that

TABLE 5-2
EPIDEMIOLOGY OF IBD

	Ulcerative colitis	Crohn's disease
Incidence (U.S.)	11/100,000	7/100,000
Age of onset	15–30 & 60–80	15–30 & 60–80
Ethnicity	Jewish > Non-Jewish Caucasian > African American > Hispanic > Asian	
Male:female ratio	1:1	1.1–1.8:1
Smoking	May prevent disease	May cause disease
Oral contraceptives	No increased risk	Relative risk 1.9
Appendectomy	Protective	Not protective
Monozygotic twins	8% concordance	67% concordance
Dizygotic twins	0% concordance	20% concordance

cover gut flora, intravenous corticosteroids, and appropriate resuscitation measures; surgery (either total proctocolectomy or subtotal colectomy) is indicated in patients who have not dramatically improved over the first 24 hours

Extraintestinal Manifestations

► Colonic disease has higher rate of extraintestinal disease than isolated small bowel disease.

► extraintestinal manifestations more common in Crohn's disease (CD) with HLA-A2, HLA-DR1, HLA-DQw5

► extraintestinal manifestations more common in UC with HLA-DR103

► Prevalence and distribution of extraintestinal manifestations:
  • musculoskeletal in 50–70%
  • rheumatologic in 15–30%
  • metabolic bone disease in 20–50%
  • dermatologic in 15%
  • ophthalmologic in 1–6%
  • GU in 4–23%

► rheumatologic:
  • peripheral arthropathy in 5–20%:
    a. *type I:* pauciarticular, < 5 joints, involving large joints, parallels bowel disease activity, acute, self-limited episodes, associated with increased incidence of erythema nodosum and uveitis, associated with HLA-B27, B35, DR103

    b.   *type II:* polyarticular, > 5 joints, involving small joints, independent of bowel disease activity, persistent symptoms, increased risk of uveitis, HLA-B44; axial arthropathy in 3–25%; ankylosing spondylitis: 5–10% of IBD patients, HLA-B27 positive, sx unrelated to underlying bowel disease, typically progressive and results in permanent skeletal damage, microscopic colitis in 60%

▶ metabolic bone disease:
- osteoporosis and osteopenia in 25–60% of IBD patients, may develop in CD even without steroid use but generally correlates with use/duration/dose of steroids, occurs early
- osteomalacia in 1–5% of CD and due to vit D deficiency
- avascular necrosis (osteonecrosis, osteochondritis desiccans) rare, increased risk with steroids + TPN

▶ dermatologic disease:
- erythema nodosum: 10–20% of IBD patients, correlates well with bowel disease activity
- pyoderma gangrenosum: 1–10% of IBD patients, ? UC > CD, independent of bowel disease activity
- Sweet's syndrome (acute febrile neutrophilic dermatosis): rare, found in both UC and CD, parallels bowel disease activity
- aphthous and angular stomatitis: most common oral lesions
- erythema multiforme: 25% of patients have CD
- psoriasis: 10% frequency in CD, HLA-A1, DR7, B17
- metastatic CD: noncaseating granulomas at extra-GI sites, most commonly skin

▶ ophthalmologic disease:
- 2–5% of UC and 3–6% of CD
- episcleritis: no loss of vision, parallels bowel disease activity
- uveitis: may progress to blindness without treatment, variable correlation with bowel disease activity but usually independent of bowel disease activity, often clusters with spondylitis/sacroiliitis and usually associated with HLA-B27

▶ hematologic disease:
- anemia: iron/B_{12} deficiency, chronic dz, Coombs-positive autoimmune hemolysis, blood loss
- autoimmune hemolytic anemia: UC > CD
- leukocytosis and thrombocytosis with active dz
- thromboembolic events: 1–39%, usually DVT or PE, UC > CD

TABLE 5-3
DIFFERENT CLINICAL, ENDOSCOPIC, AND RADIOGRAPHIC FEATURES

	Ulcerative colitis	Crohn's disease
Clinical		
Gross blood in stool	Yes	Occasionally
Mucus	Yes	Occasionally
Systemic symptoms	Occasionally	Frequently
Pain	Occasionally	Frequently
Abdominal mass	Rarely	Yes
Significant perineal disease	No	Frequently
Fistulas	No	Yes
Small intestinal obstruction	No	Frequently
Colonic obstruction	Rarely	Frequently
Response to antibiotics	No	Yes
Recurrence after surgery	No	Yes
ANCA[a]-positive	Frequently	Rarely
Endoscopic		
Rectal sparing	Rarely	Frequently
Continuous disease	Yes	Occasionally
"Cobblestoning"	No	Yes
Granuloma on biopsy	No	Occasionally
Radiographic		
Small bowel significantly abnormal	No	Yes
Abnormal terminal ileum	Occasionally	Yes
Segmental colitis	No	Yes
Asymmetrical colitis	No	Yes
Stricture	Occasionally	Frequently

[a]ANCA, antineutrophil cytoplasm antibody.

► GU disease:
  • nephrolithiasis in 7–10%, uric acid (ileostomy patients) and calcium oxalate stones (colon intact)
  • obstructive uropathy
► amyloidosis in < 1% of IBD
  • hepatobiliary disease - PSC: 2–8% of IBD, usually in males with UC, 10% incidence of cholangiocarcinoma in PSC and increased colonic dysplasia and ca in UC with PSC

Diagnosis

► **Ulcerative colitis - endoscopy:** anal involvement almost always present; evaluation with a total colonoscopy, barium enema, or biopsy is contraindicated in acute dz because of risk of perforation; hallmark is loss of vascular patterns secondary to mucosal

edema; may see mucosal erythema, contact bleeding, ulcer-
ations, or purulent exudates; **total colonoscopy:** should be performed after acute attack to determine the extent of dz; random
biopsies should be obtained; **barium enema:** can be used to
assist in diagnosis, to assess the extent of dz, and the progression of dz; benign strictures are uncommon in UC and should
be presumed malignant until proven otherwise

► **Crohn's disease - total colonoscopy** is necessary because of
rare anal involvement and skip lesions; **UGI and small bowel
follow through:** skip lesions, longitudinal ulcers, transverse
ulcers, "cobblestone" mucosa, strictures, thickening of haustral
margins, involvement of terminal ileum

Treatment

► **Ulcerative Colitis - acute phase:** hydrocortisone 100 mg Q8 hrs
for severe cases; prednisone 40–60 mg Q day tapered over
weeks for less severe cases; codeine and morphine should be
avoided as they may cause megacolon; **chronic phases:** sul-

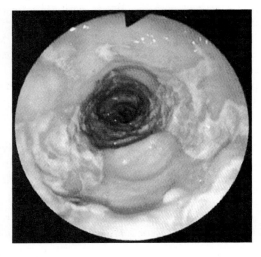

FIGURE 5-1
Crohn's colitis. (Reproduced with permission from Braunwald E, Fauci AS, Kasper DL,
et al. *Harrison's Principles of Internal Medicine.* 16th ed. McGraw-Hill, 2005.)

TABLE 5-4
INDICATIONS FOR SURGERY

Ulcerative colitis	Crohn's disease (CD)
Intractable disease	CD of small intestine
Fulminant disease	Stricture and obstruction
Toxic megacolon	unresponsive to medical therapy
Colonic perforation	Massive hemorrhage
Massive colonic hemor-	Refractory fistula
rhage	Abscess
Extracolonic disease	CD of colon and rectum
Colonic obstruction	Intractable disease
Colon cancer prophylaxis	Fulminant disease
Colon dysplasia or cancer	Perianal disease unresponsive to
	medical therapy
	Refractory fistula
	Colonic obstruction
	Cancer prophylaxis
	Colon dysplasia or cancer

fasalazine or mesalamine preparations to prolong remission; cancer surveillance (random mucosal biopsies in patients with chronic disease or disease in remission); **surgery:** indicated for intractable disease, disease present for more than 15 years, severe mucosal dysplasia, cancer, and cutaneous/systemic symptoms, DALM (dysplasia associated lesion or mass)

▶ **Crohn's disease** - hydrocortisone, prednisone, and/or sulfasalazine may be used in the acute period then tapered off as symptoms improve; in most cases, no maintenance dosing during remission; **surgery:** indicated for intractable dz, obstruction, fistulae, intra-abd abscesses, perforation, hemorrhage, cutaneous/systemic symptoms, severe anal and perianal involvement, severe mucosal dysplasia, and ca

▶ **IBD Pharmacology Pearls:**
  • Rx distribution sites:
    1. azulfidine, olsalazine (Dipentum), balsalazide - colon
    2. mesalamine (Asacol) - colon and ileum
    3. mesalamine (Pentasa) - throughout GI tract
  • combination of oral + rectal 5-ASA → ↑ efficacy in treatment of pancolitis
  • pancreatitis: may be seen with 6-MP, azathioprine, metronidazole, 5-ASA

TABLE 5-5
NEW AND EXPERIMENTAL FORMS OF THERAPY FOR IBD

Agent	Description	Rationale	Type of IBD
ISIS-2302	Antisense oligonucleotide to ICAM-1[a]	Down-regulation of ICAM-1 prevents local recruitment of white blood cells	Crohn's disease
IL[b]-10	Th2 cytokine	IL-10 suppresses production of IL-2 and IFN[c]-γ and interferes with macrophage function	Crohn's disease
IL-11	Cytokine derived from mesenchymal cells	Improves intestinal mucosal integrity	Crohn's disease
Anti-α4 antibody	Humanized antibody to α4 integrin	Antagonism of α4 integrin may prevent homing of lymphocytes to site of inflammation	Crohn's disease and ulcerative colitis
Nicotine		Possible inhibition of IL-2 and TNF[d] production; persons who quit smoking are more at risk for development of ulcerative colitis	Moderately severe ulcerative colitis
Heparin	Anticoagulant	Improvement in patients with ulcerative colitis on heparin therapy; mechanism unknown	Ulcerative colitis
Thalidomide	Immune modulator	Anti-TNF effects; inhibition of neutrophil activity	Crohn's disease
Fish oil and ω-3 fatty acids		Inhibition of leukotriene B synthesis	Crohn's disease and ulcerative colitis

[a]ICAM-1, intercellular adhesion molecule-1; [b]IL, interleukin; [c]IFN, interferon; [d]TNF, tumor necrosis factor.

- large dose, long duration of use of mesalamine may → interstitial nephritis therefore need to check u/a and creatinine q 6–12 months
- thiopurine methyltransferase (TPMT) deficiency - failure to develop therapeutic levels of 6 thioguanine (6TG) and ↑ risk of hepatotoxicity
- 6TG levels: > 230 pmol required to induce remission from use of 6-MP in IBD, > 400 pmol associated with leukopenia
- infliximab: infusion reactions seen with development of *HACA* (human anti-chimeric antibody)

REFERENCES

1. Sands BE. Therapy of inflammatory disease. *Gastroenterology* 2000; 118:S68–S82.
2. Podolsky DK. Inflammatory bowel disease. *N Engl J Med* 2002;347(6):417–429.
3. Schoon EJ, Blok BM, Geerling BJ, et al. Bone mineral density in patients with recently diagnosed inflammatory bowel disease. *Gastroenterology* 2000;119:1203–1208.
4. Lewis JD, Schwartz JS, Lichtenstein GR. Azathioprine for maintenance of remission in Crohn's disease: benefits of lymphoma. *Gastroenterology* 2000;118:1018–1024.
5. Lichtenstein GR. Treatment of fistulizing Crohn's disease. *Gastroenterology* 2000;119:1132–1147.
6. Lichtenstein GR, guest ed. Inflammatory bowel disease. In: *Gastrointestinal Endoscopy Clinics of North America.* Philadelphia: WB Saunders, July 2002.
7. Regueiro MD, guest ed. Inflammatory bowel disease. In: *Gastroenterology Clinics of North America.* Philadelphia: WB Saunders, March 2002.
8. Edwards ZC. Gastroenterology. In: Edwards TI, Mayer T, eds. *Urgent Care Medicine.* New York: McGraw-Hill, 2002:327.
9. Silverberg MS, Steinhart AH. Bone density in inflammatory bowel disease. *Clin Perspect Gastroenterol* 2000;3(3):117–124.
10. Eiden KA. Nutritional considerations in inflammatory bowel disease. *Pract Gastroenterol* 2003;XXVII(5):33–52.
11. Haens GD. Prevention of postoperative recurrence in Crohn's disease. *Inflamm Bowel Dis Monitor* 2002;4(1):12–17.
12. Bernstein CN. Dysplasia surveillance in IBD. *Inflamm Bowel Dis Monitor* 2002;4(1):18–23.
13. Watts D, Campbell S, Ghosh S. Emerging therapies in Crohn's disease. *Inflamm Bowel Dise Monitor* 2002;3(3):90–101.
14. Cullen S, Chapman R. Liver disease in IBD. *Inflamm Bowel Dis Monitor* 2002;4(2):42–48.
15. Gasche C. Anemia in IBD. *Inflamm Bowel Dis Monitor* 2002;4(2):49–55.
16. Travis S. IBD in the elderly. *Inflamm Bowel Dis Monitor* 2002;4(2):56–61.

17. Hanuaer SB, Present DH. The state of the art in the management of inflammatory bowel disease. *Rev Gastroenterological Dis* 2003;3(2):81–92.
18. Lashner BA, Kane SV. Crohn's disease treatment: safety considerations for maintenance therapy. *Gastroenterol Endoscop News* 2003;54(5):71–74.
19. Kwon JH, Farrell, RF, Peppercorn MA. Therapeutic features in inflammatory bowel disease. *Gastroenterol Endoscop News* 2002;53(4):39–43.
20. Farrell RJ, Peppercorn MA. Therapeutic features in inflammatory bowel disease. *Gastroenterol Endoscop News* 2001;52(9):33–36.
21. Sandborn WJ, Lichtenstein GR. Crohn's disease treatment algorithm: induction and maintenance of remission. *Gastroenterol Endoscop News* 2003;54(2):42–46.
22. Scherl E, Lodhavia P. Crohn's and colitis: impact of new therapies on old strategies. *Gastroenterol Endoscop News* 2003;54(7):38–42.

CHAPTER 6

GASTROINTESTINAL GENETICS PEARLS

GI GENETICS: HIGHLIGHTS
Condition-Specific Chromosomal Changes

► celiac sprue - DQA1*0501 and DQB1*0201 alleles, HLA-DR3, HLA-DQw2, HLA-DR7
► colon ca - APC (chromosome 5q21)
  • K-*ras* (codons 12, 13, and 61): seen in 50%
  • p53 (chromosome 17p13): seen in 75%
  • DCC (chromosome 18q): seen in 70%
  • MMR (*hMSH2*, *hMLH1*, hPMS1, hMPMS2): seen in 15%
► FAP - APC
► HNPCC - MHSH2, hMLH1
► acute pancreatitis - trypsinogen gene on chromosome 7, SPINK1, PRSS1, CFTR
► hemochromatosis - problem on chromosome 6: HFE gene - C282Y mutation and/or H63D mutation
► pancreatic cancer - K-*ras*, p16, BRCA2, p53, Smad4 in TGFβ
► NASH - 30% heterozygous for C282Y
► Barrett's - 13Q, p53 - 17p, 5q21
► squamous cell esophageal ca - p53, EGFR, cyclin D1
► esophageal adenocarcinoma - p53, EGFR, cyclin D1, p16, microsatellite DNA instability
► gastric adenocarcinoma - p53, microsatellite DNA instability
► small bowel lymphoma - DQA1*0501 and DQB1*0201 alleles
► PSC - HLA-DRw52a, HLA-B8
► cystic fibrosis (autosomal recessive) - CFTR gene on chromosome 7q32

► Schwachman-Diamond syndrome (autosomal recessive, exocrine pancreatic insufficiency, cyclic neutropenia) - px with chromosome 7

Serologic Markers

► celiac sprue - *EMA* (anti-endomysial antibody), *tTG* (tissue transglutaminase), *AGA* (anti-gliadin antibody), *ARA* (anti-reticulin antibody); EMA becomes negative after 6–12 months of gluten-free diet, tTG remains positive if ongoing gluten exposure present
► gastric adenocarcinoma - CA72-4
► pancreatic ca - CA19-9, K-*ras*
► small cell lung ca (may see associated intestinal pseudo-obstruction as a paraneoplastic syndrome) - antineuronal nuclear antibody (anti-Hu)

TABLE 6-1
GENES ALTERED IN SPORADIC COLORECTAL CANCER

Gene	Chromosome	Tumors with alterations (%)	Class	Function
K-ras	12	50	Proto-oncogene	Encodes guanine nucleotide-binding protein that regulates intracellular signaling
APC	5	70	Tumor suppressor	Regulation of β-catenin involved in activation of Wnt/TcF signaling (activates c-myc, cyclin D1)[a]; regulation of proliferation, apoptosis; interaction with E-cadherin (? cell adhesion)
DCC	18	70	? Tumor suppressor	Neutrin-1 receptor; caspase substrate in apoptosis; cell adhesion
SMAD4 (DPC4, MADH4)	18	?	Tumor suppressor	Nuclear transcription factor TGF-β1 signaling; regulation of angiogenesis; regulator of WAF1 promoter; downstream mediator of SMAD2
p53	17	75	Tumor suppressor	Transcription factor; regulator of cell cycle progression after cellular stress, of apoptosis, of gene expression, and of DNA repair
hMSH2	2	—[b]	DNA mismatch repair	Maintains fidelity of DNA replication
hMLH1	3	—[b]	DNA mismatch repair	Maintains fidelity of DNA replication
hMSH6	2	—[b]	DNA mismatch repair	Maintains fidelity of DNA replication
TGF-β1 RII	3	—[c]	Tumor suppressor	Receptor for signaling in the TGF-β1 pathway; inhibitor of colonic epithelial proliferation, often mutated in tumors with MSI

[a]β-Catenin mutations (downstream of APC) are found in 16–25% of microsatellite instability (MSI) colon cancers, but not in microsatellite stable (MSS) cancers.
[b]Approximately 15% of sporadic colorectal cancers demonstrate MSI associated with alterations in mismatch repair genes (principally hMSH2 and hMLH1 but also hMSH3, hMSH6, hPMS1, and hPMS2).
[c]Mutated in 73–90% of MSI colon cancers. Up to 55% of MSS colon cancer cell lines may demonstrate a TGF-β signaling blockage distal to TGF-β1 RII.

TABLE 6-2
INTERPRETATION OF GENETIC TESTING FOR HEMOCHROMATOSIS

C282Y homozygote
This is the classic genetic pattern that is seen in > 90% of typical cases.
Expression of disease ranges from no evidence of iron overload to
massive iron overload with organ dysfunction. Siblings have approximately a one in four chance of being affected and should have genetic
testing. For children to be affected, the other parent must be at least a
heterozygote. If iron studies are normal, false-positive genetic testing
or a nonexpressing homozygote should be considered.

C282Y/H63D - Compound heterozygote
This patient carries one copy of the major mutation and one copy of the
minor mutation. Most patients with this genetic pattern have normal
iron studies. A small percentage of compound heterozygotes have
been found to have mild to moderate iron overload. Severe iron overload is usually seen in the setting of another concomitant risk factor
(alcoholism, viral hepatitis).

C282Y heterozygote
This patient carries one copy of the major mutation. This pattern is seen
in about 10% of the white population and is usually associated with
normal iron studies. In rare cases, the iron studies are high in the
range expected in a homozygote rather than a heterozygote. These
cases may carry an unknown hemochromatosis mutation and liver
biopsy is helpful to determine the need for venesection therapy.

H63D homozygote
This patient carries two copies of the minor mutation. Most patients
with this genetic pattern have normal iron studies. A small percentage
of these cases have been found to have mild to moderate iron overload. Severe iron overload is usually seen in the setting of another
concomitant risk factor (alcoholism, viral hepatitis).

H63D heterozygote
This patient carries one copy of the minor mutation. This pattern is seen
in about 20% of the white population and is usually associated with
normal iron studies. This pattern is so common in the general population that the presence of iron overload may be related to another risk
factor. Liver biopsy may be required to determine the cause of the
iron overload and the need for treatment in these cases.

No HFE mutations
Iron overload has been described in families with mutations in other
iron-related genes (transferrin receptor 2 and IREG1). Other hemochromatosis mutations will likely be discovered in the future. If iron
overload is present without any HFE mutations, a careful history for
other risk factors must be reviewed and liver biopsy may be useful to
determine the cause of the iron overload and the need for treatment.
Most of these are isolated, nonfamilial cases.

REFERENCES

1. Friedman SL, McQuaid KR, Grendell JH. *Diagnosis & Treatment in Gastroenterology.* New York: Lange Medical Books/McGraw-Hill, 2003.
2. Braunwald E, Fauci AS, Kasper DL, et al. *Harrison's Principles of Internal Medicine.* 15th ed. New York: McGraw-Hill, 2001.
3. Bowlus CL. Genetic testing in hemochromatosis. *Pract Gastroenterol* 2001;XXV(9):44–56.
4. Sweeney JT, Ulrich CD. Genetics of pancreatic disease. *Clin Perspect Gastroenterol* 2002;5(2):110–116.
5. Feldman M, Scharschmidt BF, Sleisenger MH. *Sleisenger & Fordtran's Gastrointestinal and Liver Disease.* 6th ed. Philadelphia: WB Saunders, 1998.
6. Yamada Y, ed. *Textbook of Gastroenterology.* 3rd ed. Philadelphia: Lippincott Williams & Wilkins, 1999.
7. Goldman L, Bennett JC, eds. *Cecil Textbook of Medicine.* 21st ed. Philadelphia: WB Saunders, 2000.
8. Ahlquist DA, guest ed. Colorectal cancer prevention and detection. In: *Gastroenterology Clinics of North America* 2002;31(4):926–1181. Philadelphia: WB Saunders, 2002.
9. Lichtenstein GR, guest ed. Inflammatory bowel disease. In: *Gastrointestinal Endoscopy Clinics of North America* 2002;12(3):433–646. Philadelphia: WB Saunders, 2002.
10. Schuppan D. Current concepts of celiac disease pathogenesis. *Gastroenterology* 2000;119:234–242.
11. Jarvinen HJ, Aarnio M, Mustonen H, et al. Controlled 15-year trial on screening for colorectal cancer in families with hereditary nonpolyposis colorectal cancer. *Gastroenterology* 2000;118:829–834.
12. El-Serag HB, Inadomi JM, Kowdley KV. Screening for hereditary hemochromatosis in siblings and children of affected patients. *Ann Intern Med* 2000;132:261–269.
13. Bonen DK, Cho JH. The genetics of inflammatory bowel disease. *Gastroenterology* 2003;124:521–536.
14. Winawer S, Fletcher R, Rex D, et al. Colorectal cancer screening and surveillance: clinical guidelines and rationale—update based on new evidence. *Gastroenterology* 2003;124:544–560.
15. Grady WM. Genetic testing for high-risk colon cancer patients. *Gastroenterology* 2003;124:1574–1594.
16. Calvert PM, Frucht H. The genetics of colorectal cancer. *Ann Intern Med* 2002;137:603–612.
17. Chung DC, Rustgi AK. The hereditary nonpolyposis colorectal cancer syndrome: genetics and clinical implications. *Ann Intern Med* 2003;138:560–570.

CHAPTER 7

GASTROINTESTINAL BLEEDING

GASTROINTESTINAL BLEEDING
Highlights

► **Major Syndromes:**
  - upper GI bleed (UGIB): acid-peptic disease, vascular lesions (varices; gastric antral vascular ectasia (GAVE); Dieulafoy's lesion; AVMs), cancer, medication (NSAIDs, steroids, aspirin) and alcohol-induced lesions, Mallory-Weiss tear
  - lower GI bleed (LGIB): diverticular disease, colitides (IBD, ischemic bowel disease, radiation colitis), vascular lesions (hemorrhoids, AVMs), cancer
  - occult/obscure: hemobilia, hemosuccus pancreaticus, AVMs, GAVE, blue rubber bleb nevus syndrome, Meckel's diverticulum, aortoenteric fistula

► UGIB may often present as coffee-ground emesis, hematemesis, or melenic stool, while LGIB will often manifest as *BRBPR* (bright red blood per rectum), maroon or burgundy colored fecal material, or blood clots per rectum.

► at least 100 mL of blood required to produce a melenic stool

► Orthostasis implies a ≥ 10% depletion in intravascular volume. The presence of shock indicates a loss of at least 20–25% intravascular volume.

► Risk factors for increased mortality from UGIB include age > 60, the presence of co-morbid conditions such as cardiac, renal, or liver disease, portal hypertension, and visible vessel on endoscopy.

► Risk factors for recurrent UGIB include use of tobacco, alcohol, anticoagulant medication or ASA/NSAID, and thrombocytopenia.

► UGI tract sources are the etiology of two-thirds of cases of GI bleeding.

TABLE 7-1
CAUSES OF SEVERE UPPER GI BLEEDING[a]

Diagnosis	Number of patients (%) ($n = 948$)
Peptic ulcers	524 (55)
Gastroesophageal varices	131 (14)
Angiomas	54 (6)
Mallory-Weiss tear	45 (5)
Tumors	42 (4)
Erosions	41 (4)
Dieulafoy's lesion	6 (1)
Other	105 (11)

[a]Data from the Center for Ulcer Research and Education (CURE) Hemostasis Research Group, UCLA School of Medicine and the West Los Angeles VA Medical Center.

UGI Hemorrhage

▶ **Acid-peptic disease** - includes bleeding related to esophagitis, gastritis, and frank ulcer disease; symptoms may vary from an asymptomatic state to heartburn, abd pain, dysphagia; most common cause of severe UGI hemorrhage; lab abnormalities include ↓ Hb/Hct and elevated BUN and creatinine; endoscopy

TABLE 7-2
ETIOLOGY OF ACUTE LOWER GI BLEEDING

Common conditions
 Colonic diverticulosis
 Angiodysplasia
 Neoplasia (polyps and cancer)
 Colitis (idiopathic, infectious, and ischemic)
 Anorectal lesions (hemorrhoids, anal fissures, and idiopathic rectal
  ulcers)
Less common conditions
 Postpolypectomy bleeding
 Radiation-related injury
 Endometriosis
 Vasculitis
 Upper GI bleeding manifesting as hemochezia
Rare conditions
 Aortoenteric fistula
 GI bleeding in athletes
 Meckel's diverticulum
 Small-bowel diverticular bleeding
 Colonic varices and portal colopathy
 Dieulafoy's lesion of the colon
 Intussusception

is diagnostic method of choice; medical tx regimens include H2 blocker therapy, and proton pump inhibitors (PPIs); eradication of *Helicobacter pylori* is indicated for those who test positive; endoscopic intervention may include injection therapy or thermal coagulation for those patients with persistent or recurrent bleeding from a visible vessel

▶ **Varices** - may commonly see sequelae of underlying liver disease including encephalopathy, jaundice, palmar erythema, spider telangiectasia, ascites; ↓ Hb/Hct and platelets, elevated LFTs and PT/PTT, ↓ albumin and cholesterol; endoscopy is diagnostic and therapeutic method of choice; endoscopic tx includes injection sclerotherapy and band ligation; for those patients refractory to an endoscopic approach, options include *TIPS* (transjugular intrahepatic portosystemic shunt) and surgical intervention

▶ **Dieulafoy's lesion** - dilated aberrant submucosal vessel with bleeding due to erosion of overlying epithelium; usually located along the high lesser curvature; often presents as recurrent massive bleeding, with dx sometimes elusive to make due to absence of active bleeding at time of endoscopy or large volume of blood in the stomach making visualization difficult; endoscopy with thermal coagulation via heater probe or multipolar electrocoagulation is tx of choice with surgical wedge resection indicated in those cases that fail to respond to an endoscopic approach

▶ **Miscellaneous vascular lesions** - includes AVMs and GAVE ("watermelon stomach"); often present as chronic, intermittent bleeds; often see iron-deficiency anemia and need for repeat transfusions; endoscopy is diagnostic method of choice

▶ **Medication-induced lesions** - increased risk in patients taking ASA/NSAIDs, steroids, iron, potassium, and certain antibiotics (e.g., doxycycline and tetracycline); endoscopy is diagnostic method of choice; tx includes discontinuation of the offending agent and a course of H2 blockers, PPIs, and sucralfate when indicated

▶ **Mallory-Weiss tear** - located in the distal esophagus and induced by forceful retching or vomiting; patients with portal hypertension at increased risk; presents with hematemesis; endoscopy is diagnostic method of choice; bleeding usually resolves spontaneously without tx; when bleeding is active and/or persistent, tx options include endoscopic injection or thermal coagulation

Lower GI Hemorrhage

▶ **Diverticular bleed** - history of LGIB with passage of burgundy or maroon stools and/or more blood than fecal material; ↓ Hb/Hct; bleeding usually resolves spontaneously; diagnostic techniques include colonoscopy, radionuclide red cell scan, and angiography; tx options in patients with persistent, massive, or recurrent bleeding include angiographic embolization or vasopressin infusion, endoscopic injection/thermal coagulation/electrocoagulation, or surgical resection depending on the degree of bleeding, the clinical condition of the patient, and the ability to pinpoint to the site of bleeding

▶ **Colitides** - includes IBD, radiation colitis, ischemic colitis, and infectious colitis; presentation and tx dependent on the etiology of the colitis; lab abnormalities may include ↓ Hb/Hct, iron-deficiency anemia, elevated WBC, abnormal stool studies; diagnostic approach is also dependent on suspected etiology and may include colonoscopy, radiologic imaging, and stool studies

▶ **Hemorrhoids** - usually presents as BRBPR, though on occasion may present as an iron-deficiency anemia; bleeding usually painless; diagnostic symptoms may include rectal pruritus, constipation with straining, and hemorrhoidal prolapse; dx may be made via anoscopy or flexible sigmoidoscopy; tx options include local comfort measures, sitz baths, band ligation, and surgical intervention depending on the severity of the hemorrhoids

Occult/Obscure GI Hemorrhage

▶ **AVMs** - often the etiology of occult/obscure GI bleeding; often see iron-deficiency anemia with need for recurrent transfusion; may see intermittent episodes of hematochezia; colonoscopy and angiographic approaches are diagnostic methods of choice

▶ **Hemosuccus pancreaticus** - results from bleeding from peripancreatic vessels into the pancreatic duct usually as a result of chronic pancreatitis which may be related to a pseudocyst or pseudoaneurysm; endoscopy accompanied by a high degree of suspicion in the appropriate clinical setting often leads to dx, but angiography may be required; tx options include angiographic embolization and surgery

▶ **Hemobilia** - bleeding due to hemorrhage into the biliary tract most commonly related to trauma; bleeding may also be related to neoplasm, cholelithiasis, aneurysm; endoscopy accompanied by a high degree of suspicion in the appropriate clinical setting often leads to dx but angiography may be required; tx options include angiographic embolization and surgery

▶ **Meckel's diverticulum** - congenital anomaly in which there is incomplete obliteration of the vitelline duct; seen in up to 2% of the general population and most common cause of GI bleeding in children; diverticulum often lined with gastric mucosa and usually located within 100 cm of the ileocecal valve; may present with "currant jelly" stools or melena; dx is usually via a Meckel's technetium scan; tx is surgical resection of the diverticulum

TABLE 7-3
ETIOLOGY OF GI BLEEDING

Etiology of UGI bleed	% of bleeds	Comments
Peptic ulcer disease	50%	Mortality rate up to 25%; 20–25% rebleeding rate
Varices	10–20%	Mortality rate up to 40% during hospitalization and 60–80% at 4 years; 50% rebleeding rate if untreated
Portal hypertensive gastropathy	20% of cases in cirrhotic patients	
Mallory-Weiss tear	5–10%	< 10% rebleeding rate
AVMs	5–10%	
Peptic "-itides," e.g., gastritis, esophagitis	< 5%	
Neoplasm	1%	
Other	10%	Includes hemobilia, aortoenteric fistula, Dieulafoy's lesion, hemosuccus pancreaticus

Etiology of LGI bleed	% of bleeds	Comments
Diverticulosis	up to 55%	Up to 40% rebleeding rate
AVMs	up to 10%	
Colorectal neoplasm	up to 25%	
Colitides	up to 20%	
Hemorrhoids	up to 10%	
Other	up to 10%	Includes postpolypectomy bleed, Meckel's diverticulum, colonic varices

REFERENCES

1. Edwards ZC. Gastroenterology. In: Edwards TI, Mayer T, eds. *Urgent Care Medicine*. New York: McGraw-Hill, 2002:327.
2. SL Friedman, KR McQuaid, JH Grendell. *Diagnosis & Treatment in Gastroenterology*. New York: Lange Medical Books/McGraw-Hill, 2003.
3. Edmundowicz SA. *20 Common Problems in Gastroenterology*. New York: McGraw-Hill, 2002.
4. Tierney LM, McPhee SJ, Papadakis MA. *Current Medical Diagnosis and Treatment*. New York: McGraw-Hill, 2003.

CHAPTER 8

DIVERTICULAR DISEASE

DIVERTICULAR DISEASE
Highlights

▶ **Major Syndromes:**
  - diverticulitis
  - diverticular bleed

▶ Diverticulitis and diverticular bleeding rarely present concomitantly.

▶ Patients tend to be older adults who have had similar bouts in the past.

▶ Diverticular bleeding develops in 5–10% of patients with diverticular disease and accounts for up to 50% of cases of lower GI bleeding (LGIB) in general.

▶ Bleeding ceases spontaneously in up to 90% of the cases of diverticular hemorrhage.

Symptoms/Signs/Labs

▶ **Diverticulitis** - typical presentation of abd pain (most often in lower quadrants, L > R), change in bowel habits (diarrhea or constipation), and fever; N&V suggests ileus or obstruction, may also have complaint of tenesmus and/or urinary frequency; abd pain on palpation (generally LLQ), may also see voluntary guarding, rebound, or inflammatory mass and left-sided tenderness on rectal exam; elevated WBC with left shift on differential, radiologic imaging may reveal evidence of ileus, obstruction, or perforation depending on the severity of the episode; potential complications include peritonitis, sepsis, fistulous disease, ileus, and bowel obstruction

▶ **Diverticular bleed** - history of LGIB with passage of burgundy or maroon stools and/or clots; diarrhea with more blood than fecal material; orthostasis and tachycardia if intravascular volume is depleted; Hg/Hct may be normal to low depending on the degree of bleeding and the timing of presentation; abd exam may be unremarkable, rectal examination consistent with non-hemorrhoidal GI bleeding

Diagnosis

▶ **Diverticulitis** - physical exam and laboratory evaluation, air-fluid levels on plain film in obstruction and free air in perforation; CT scan → inflammation, thickened bowel wall, phlegmon, fatty infiltration, and abscess depending on severity of acute episode

▶ **Diverticular bleed** - history of LGIB with passage of burgundy or maroon stools and/or clots; diarrhea with more blood than fecal material; orthostasis and tachycardia if intravascular volume is depleted; Hg/Hct may be normal to low depending on the degree of bleeding and the timing of presentation; abd exam may be unremarkable, rectal examination consistent with non-hemorrhoidal GI bleeding; red cell scan (able to detect bleeding rate as low as 0.1 mL/minute), angiogram if bleeding is active and at a rate > 0.5 mL/minute; colonoscopy → difficult to perform acutely but may see active bleeding site, reaccumulation of blood or adherent clot at a specific site despite irrigation, inflamed mucosa

Treatment

▶ **Diverticulitis** - if mild to moderate bout without evidence of systemic toxicity, may treat as outpatient with close F/U with a 7–10-day course of a broad-spectrum abx regimen and instructions to maintain a low-fiber diet during the acute episode; IV abx, hospitalization, and surgery may be required depending on the presentation or progression of the patient's clinical condition physical exam and laboratory evaluation, air-fluid levels on plain film in obstruction, and free air in perforation.

▶ **Diverticular bleed** - hemodynamic resuscitation and supportive care, including blood transfusion will be sufficient in most cases as bleeding generally resolves spontaneously with an initial episode (25% risk of re-bleeding, increasing to 50% with a subsequent episode); angiographic embolization and/or surgical resection of the affected colonic segment may be required if persistent or recurrent bleeding occurs.

REFERENCES

1. Edwards ZC. Gastroenterology. In: Edwards TI, Mayer T, eds. *Urgent Care Medicine.* New York: McGraw-Hill, 2002:327.
2. Friedman SL, McQuaid KR, Grendell JH. *Diagnosis & Treatment in Gastroenterology.* New York: Lange Medical Books/McGraw-Hill, 2003.
3. Goldman L, Bennett JC, eds. *Cecil Textbook of Medicine.* 21st ed. Philadelphia: WB Saunders, 2000.
4. Bland KI. *The Practice of General Surgery.* Philadelphia: WB Saunders, 2002.

PART II

THE LIVER AND BILIARY TREE

CHAPTER 9

HEPATITIDES

VIRAL HEPATITIS
Highlights

► **Helpful in differentiating syndromes:**
- serology and lab profile
- symptoms and demographics
- incubation period
- mode of transmission

► **Major Syndromes:**
- hepatitis A (HAV)
- hepatitis B (HBV)
- hepatitis C (HCV)
- hepatitis D (HDV)
- hepatitis E (HEV)

► sexual transmission: HBV >> HDV > HCV > HAV > HEV

Demographics

► **Hepatitis A** - RNA virus; incubation: 15–45 days; transmission: oral-fecal (water, food, contact); highest attack rate in late childhood (ages 5–14); fulminant hepatitis rare and more common in older ages or in patients with underlying liver dz

► **Hepatitis B** - DNA virus; incubation: 4 weeks–6 months; transmission: parenteral, including sexual contact (30% transmission rate); worldwide - 350 million carriers (1 million in U.S.), 2 billion infected; accounts for 15% of chronic liver dz cases; increased risk for HCC in chronic dz; conversion to chronic dz decreases with age (100% in infants, 70% in childhood, 5% in healthy adults); chronic - persistence of HBsAg for ≥ 6 months (highest risk in neonates born to HBV carrier who is HBeAg + and has high level of HBV DNA)

▶ **Hepatitis C** - RNA virus (6 viral genotypes, with genotypes 1, 2, and 3 seen in U.S., genotype 1 more common in blacks and less responsive to therapy); incubation: 3–12 weeks; transmission: parenteral and community (3% transmission rate); most common cause of viral hepatitis in U.S.; 55–85% of acute cases progress to chronic dz; accounts for 40% of transplant cases and 40% of CLD patients; usually clinically silent for ≥ 20 years; predictors of rapid dz progression - concomitant ETOH, HIV, or HBV co-infection, older age at time of HCV acquisition, immunosuppressed state, hemochromatosis

▶ **Hepatitis D** - RNA virus; incubation: 3 weeks–5 months; transmission: parenteral, including sexual contact; limited to patients with concurrent persistent HBV infection; may occur coincident with HBV acute infection or as superinfection in chronic HBV infection: co-infection causes severe acute dz but low risk of chronic infection; super-infection usually results in chronic HDV and increases risk of severe chronic liver dz

▶ **Hepatitis E** - RNA virus; incubation: 2–9 weeks; transmission: fecal-oral (water, food, contact); occurs in endemic areas with poor sanitary conditions and with sporadic transmission among children; highest attack rate age 15–40; 20% case fatality rate in pregnant women; no chronic dz state

Symptoms/Signs/Labs

General

▶ **Acute** - nonspecific, fatigue, anorexia, malaise, nausea, low-grade fever, arthralgias, dark urine, pruritus, scleral icterus, jaundice, elevated AST/ALT: often > 1000 and ALT > AST

▶ **Chronic** - typically asxtic until signs/symptoms of advanced liver dz develop

▶ **Hepatitis A** - often asxtic

▶ **Hepatitis B** - associated extrahepatic disorders: polyarteritis nodosa (rare but 30–35% case fatality rate), renal dz: membranous glomerulonephritis - seen primarily in children, minimal change dz, IgA nephropathy, vasculitic glomerulonephritis;

TABLE 9-1
CLINICAL AND EPIDEMIOLOGIC FEATURES OF VIRAL HEPATITIS

Feature	HAV	HBV	HCV	HDV	HEV
Incubation (days)	15–45, mean 30	30–180, mean 60–90	15–160, mean 50	30–180, mean 60–90	14–60, mean 40
Onset	Acute	Insidious or acute	Insidious	Insidious or acute	Acute
Age preference	Children, young adults	Young adults (sexual and percutaneous), babies, toddlers	Any age, but more common in adults	Any age (similar to HBV)	Young adults (20–40 years)
Transmission					
Fecal-oral	+++	—	—	—	+++
Percutaneous	Unusual	+++	+++	+++	—
Perinatal	—	+++	±[a]	+	—
Sexual	±	++	±[a]	++	—
Clinical					
Severity	Mild	Occasionally severe	Moderate	Occasionally severe	Mild
Fulminant	0.1%	0.1–1%	0.1%	5–20%[b]	1–2%[e]
Progression to chronicity	None	Occasional (1–10%) (90% of neonates)	Common (50–70% chronic hepatitis; 80–90% chronic infection)	Common[d]	None
Carrier	None	0.1–30%[c]	1.5–3.2%	Variable[f]	None
Cancer	None	+ (neonatal infection)	+	±	None
Prognosis	Excellent	Worse with age, debility	Moderate	Acute, good Chronic, poor	Good

continued

TABLE 9-1
CLINICAL AND EPIDEMIOLOGIC FEATURES OF VIRAL HEPATITIS (CONTINUED)

Feature	HAV	HBV	HCV	HDV	HEV
Prophylaxis	IG Inactivated vaccine	HBIG Recombinant vaccine	None	HBV vaccine (none for HBV carriers)	Unknown
Therapy	None	Interferon Lamivudine	Interferon plus ribavirin	Interferon ±	None

[a]Primarily with HIV co-infection and high-level viremia in index case; risk approximately 5%.

[b]Up to 5% in acute HBV/HDV co-infection; up to 20% in HDV superinfection of chronic HBV infection.

[c]Varies considerably throughout the world and in subpopulations within countries.

[d]In Acute HBV/HDV co-infection, the frequency of chronicity is the same as that for HBV; in HDV superinfection, chronicity is invariable.

[e]10–20% in pregnant women.

[f]Common in Mediterranean countries, rare in North America and western Europe.

pre-core mutant - HBsAg and HBV DNA positive with negative HBeAg, may be asxtic carrier or have progressive severe dz

- *asymptomatic carrier:*
  - HBsAg positive with normal AST and ALT
  - most HBeAg and HBV DNA negative
  - spontaneous clearance of HBsAg 1% per year
  - appears not to have increased risk for HCC
- *chronic:*
  - HBsAg + HBeAg + HBV DNA positive
  - elevated AST and ALT
  - necroinflammatory dz on liver bx
  - 10% spontaneous loss of HBeAg and/or HBV DNA per year and 0.5% clearance of HBsAg per year with consequent reduction of risk of development of cirrhosis
  - 12% per year risk of development of cirrhosis
  - 6% per year risk of progression from cirrhosis to decompensated dz
  - 2.5% risk of development of HCC in cirrhotic

▶ **Hepatitis C** - extrahepatic disorders: cryoglobulinemia (immune complex vasculitis associated with joint, skin, and kidney involvement), glomerulonephritis

- *chronic:*
  - 0.1–7% annual progression to cirrhosis
  - 3–7% annual progression from cirrhosis to decompensated liver dz
  - 1–4% progression from cirrhosis to HCC (and usually not seen until 30 years of dz)
  - moderate to severe necroinflammatory activity and/or fibrosis with progression to cirrhosis in 10 years
  - cirrhosis in HCV → 80% 10-year survival rate
  - cirrhosis in HCV with complications → 50% mortality rate over 5 years
  - HCV antibody and HCV RNA positive and elevated AST and ALT

Diagnosis

▶ **Hepatitis A** - acute: anti-HAV IgM positive; anti-HAV-IgM appears early and generally lasts 3–6 months. Anti-HAV IgG appears and persists for life after acute infection.

▶ **Hepatitis B** - HBsAg positivity establishes diagnosis, appears about 6 weeks after infection, and usually cleared within 3 months in transient dz. Anti-HBcIgM positivity implies acute or reactivated infection. Anti-HBsAg positivity is generally detectable 3 months after infection and infers recovery and immunity. HBsAg implies infection. HBeAg and HBV DNA imply HBV replication.

▶ **Hepatitis C** - anti-HCV antibody, positive viral RNA, positive recombinant immunoblot assay (RIBA)

▶ **Hepatitis D** - HBsAg plus HDV antibody positive

▶ **Hepatitis E** - serologic marker: anti-HEV (indicates current or past infection, anti-HEV IgM indicates current or recent infection)

Treatment

▶ **Hepatitis A**
   1. HAV vaccine:
      - 90% immunity
      - effective for pre-exposure prophylaxis
      - provides protection for 10 years
   2. Immune globulin:
      - effective post-exposure
      - recommended for household and sexual contacts within 2 weeks of exposure

▶ **Hepatitis B**
   1. *General* - avoid ETOH and get HAV vaccine
   2. *Asymptomatic carrier* - no addn'l treatment
   3. HBV vaccine:
      - given at 0, 1, and 6 months
      - protects for 5 years
      - pre-exposure prophylaxis; post-exposure prophylaxis when combined with HBIG
      - double-dose recommended for dialysis patients
      - dialysis, ESLD, and immunocompromised less responsive
   4. *Chronic disease* - treatment response = RNA < 50 IU/mL or > 2 logarithmic decline
      a. interferon alfa-2b at 10 mm units tiw × 4 months or 5 mm units daily × 4 months, with goal of loss of HBeAg and HBV DNA:
         - 35–45% response rate
         - 5–10% relapse rate in 1st year and will require re-tx

TABLE 9-2
LABORATORY EVALUATION—HEPATITIS

	Hepatitis A		
	Hep A antigen	IgM Hep A antibody	Total Hep A antibody
Acute			
Early	+++	+++	+++
Late	−	+	+++
Recovery	−	−	+++
Transmission	Enteric		
	Can be from blood or body fluids (rarely)		
Incubation	15–50 days		

	Hepatitis B					
	Hep B s antigen	Hep B s antibody	Hep B c antigen IgM	Hep B c antigen IgG	Hep B e antigen	Hep B e antibody
Acute	+	−	+	−	±	±
Chronic	+	−	±	+	±	±
Chronic carrier	+	−	±	+	−	±
Transmission	Blood					
	Body fluids (semen, saliva, blood)					
	Enteric					
Incubation	45–160 days					

continued

TABLE 9-2
LABORATORY EVALUATION—HEPATITIS (CONTINUED)

	Hep C antibody	RIBA	Viral RNA
			Hepatitis C
Acute	±	±	+
Chronic	+	+	+
Transmission	Blood		
	Sexual transmission is possible		
Incubation	15–160 days		

TABLE 9-3
LIVER TEST PATTERNS IN HEPATOBILIARY DISORDERS

Type of disorder	Bilirubin	Aminotransferases	Alkaline phosphatase	Albumin	Prothrombin time
Hemolysis/Gilbert syndrome	Normal to 5 mg/dL 85% due to indirect fractions No bilirubinuria	Normal	Normal	Normal	Normal
Acute hepatocellular necrosis (viral and drug hepatitis, hepatotoxins, acute heart failure)	Both fractions may be elevated Peak usually follows aminotransferases Bilirubinuria	Elevated, often > 500 IU ALT > AST	Normal to < 3 × normal elevation	Normal	Usually normal. If > 5 × above control and not corrected by parenteral vitamin K, suggests poor prognosis
Chronic hepatocellular disorders	Both fractions may be elevated Bilirubinuria	Elevated, but usually < 300 IU	Normal to < 3 × normal elevation	Often decreased	Often prolonged Fails to correct with parenteral vitamin K
Alcoholic hepatitis Cirrhosis	Both fractions may be elevated Bilirubinuria	AST:ALT >2 suggests alcoholic hepatitis or cirrhosis	Normal to < 3 × normal elevation	Often decreased	Often prolonged Fails to correct with parenteral vitamin K

continued

TABLE 9-3
LIVER TEST PATTERNS IN HEPATOBILIARY DISORDERS (CONTINUED)

Type of disorder	Bilirubin	Aminotransferases	Alkaline phosphatase	Albumin	Prothrombin time
Intra- and extrahepatic cholestasis	Both fractions may be elevated	Normal to moderate elevation	Elevated, often >4× normal elevation	Normal, unless chronic	Normal
(Obstructive jaundice)	Bilirubinuria	Rarely > 500 IU			If prolonged, will correct with parenteral vitamin K
Infiltrative diseases (tumor, granulomata); partial bile duct obstruction	Usually normal	Normal to slight elevation	Elevated, often >4× normal elevation Fractionate, or confirm liver origin with 5′ nucleotidase or gamma glutamyl transpeptidase	Normal	Normal

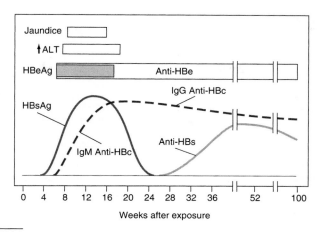

FIGURE 9-1

Lab features of acute hepatitis B. (Reproduced with permission from Braunwald E, Fauci AS, Kasper DL, et al. *Harrison's Principles of Internal Medicine.* 16th ed. McGraw-Hill, 2005.)

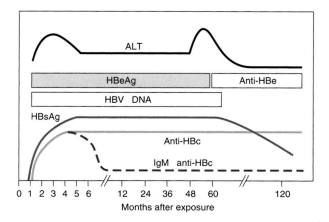

FIGURE 9-2

Lab features of chronic hepatitis B. (Reproduced with permission from Braunwald E, Fauci AS, Kasper DL, et al. *Harrison's Principles of Internal Medicine.* 16th ed. McGraw-Hill, 2005.)

TABLE 9-4
SIMPLIFIED DIAGNOSTIC APPROACH IN PATIENTS PRESENTING WITH ACUTE HEPATITIS

| | Serologic tests of patient's serum | | | |
HBsAg	IgM anti-HAV	IgM anti-HBc	Anti-HCV	Diagnostic interpretation
+	−	+	−	Acute hepatitis B
+	−	−	−	Chronic hepatitis B
+	+	−	−	Acute hepatitis A super-imposed on chronic hepatitis B
+	+	+	−	Acute hepatitis A and B
−	+	−	−	Acute hepatitis A
−	+	+	−	Acute hepatitis A and B (HBsAg below detection threshold)
−	−	+	−	Acute hepatitis B (HBsAg below detection threshold)
−	−	−	+	Acute hepatitis C

- 70–80% responders with flare characterized by elevation in AST and ALT at weeks 4–8 of therapy (may see ↑ to 1000); if accompanied by jaundice or deterioration in synthetic fxn, reduce dose or discontinue therapy
- side effects: flulike syndrome in 98%, depression, irritability
- reduce/discontinue therapy: severe granulocytopenia or thrombocytopenia
- positive predictors of response: high ALT, low HBV DNA levels, active necroinflammatory lesions on bx, female, negative HDV, HBV acquired after neonatal period, short duration of dz prior to tx, absence of immunosuppressive dz or therapies
- should not be used in decompensated cirrhosis but low dose (0.5–1 mm units daily) can be considered in Child's A or Child's B

  b. lamivudine:
- 100 mg q day
- reduce dose if creatinine clearance < 50

TABLE 9-5
CLINICAL AND LABORATORY FEATURES OF CHRONIC HEPATITIS

Type of hepatitis	Diagnostic test(s)	Autoantibodies	Therapy
Chronic hepatitis B	HBsAg, IgG, anti-HBc, HBeAg, HBV DNA	Uncommon	INF-α, lamivudine
Chronic hepatitis C	Anti-HCV (EIA and RIBA), HCV RNA	Anti-LKM1[a]	INF-α plus ribavirin
Chronic hepatitis D	Anti-HDV, HDV RNA, HBsAg, IgG, anti-HBc	Anti-LKM3	INF-α (?)
Autoimmune hepatitis	ANA[b] (homogeneous), anti-LKM1(±), hyperglobulinemia	ANA, anti-LKM1, anti-SLA[c]	Prednisone, azathioprine
Drug-associated	—	Uncommon	Withdraw drug
Cryptogenic	All negative	None	Prednisone (?), azathioprine (?)

[a]Antibodies to liver-kidney microsomes type I (autoimmune hepatitis type II and some cases of hepatitis C).
[b]Antinuclear antibody (autoimmune hepatitis type I).
[c]Antibodies to soluble liver antigen (autoimmune hepatitis type III).
NOTE: HBsAg, hepatitis B surface antigen; EIA, enzyme immunoassay; RIBA, recombinant immunoblot assay; INF-α, interferon α.

- inhibitor of HBV reverse transcription
- 15–50% of patients develop YMDD mutant after 1–3 years of therapy
- useful in helping to prevent recurrent HBV posttransplant
- ? duration of treatment of 1 year

5. *Liver transplantation* - high frequency of recurrent HBV infection in grafted liver
6. *HCC* - small, unresectable tumor (≤5 cm) or no more than 3 tumors with each ≤3 cm has 4-year survival rate with transplantation

▶ **Hepatitis C**
   1. *General* - avoid ETOH and get HAV and HBV vaccines

2. *Chronic*:
   a. interferon monotherapy:
      - should be limited to those who can not be tx'd with combination therapy
      - indications: anti-HCV positive plus elevated ALT plus detectable HCV RNA plus evidence of chronic hepatitis on bx
      - 3 MU tiw × 12 months: 10%–20% sustained response rate
      - lack of response at 3 months implies nonresponder
      - positive predictors of response: shorter duration of dz, younger age, milder histologic features, lower levels of HCV RNA, genotypes 2 and 3, limited quasispecies diversity
      - factors that decrease response rate: increased age, increased duration of dz, increased HCV RNA levels, increased histologic stage, genotype 1b, increased iron load, presence of quasispecies
   b. interferon + ribavirin - therapy of choice:
      - interferon in conventional doses + ribavirin 1000–1200 mg q day for 6–12 months
      - genotype 1: response rate of 16% rate at 6 months and 28% at 12 months
      - genotypes 2 and 3: response rate of 31% at 6 months and 38% at 12 months; 60–70% sustained response rate
      - better response rate in female, age < 40, viral load < 1 mm IU/mL
      - genotypes 1 and 4 less responsive to therapy
      - ribavirin side effects: hemolytic anemia
      - contraindicated in impaired renal function, chronic anemia
      - discontinuation of therapy necessary in 20% but if for < 2 weeks has no adverse effect on response rate
   c. pegylated interferon alfa-2b:
      - approved as monotherapy as once-weekly injection at 1.5 µg/kg
      - efficacy similar to combination therapy
      - combination with ribavirin @ > 10.6 mg/kg results in 45% response rate in genotype 1 and 90% response rate in genotypes 2 and 3

   d. liver transplantation:
      - invariable recurrence of HCV infection but < 50% with allograft damage and infection generally mild, clinically silent, and rarely progresses to hepatic failure
      - 5-year survival similar to that in patients with other indications for transplant

► **Hepatitis D**
   - alfa-interferon in same doses as HBV therapy (50% response rate and relapse common)

► **Hepatitis E**
   - supportive care; no chronic dz state

ETOH Hepatitis

► acute ETOH hepatitis: 10–20% mortality rate
► abstinence → 38% cirrhosis, 52% steatohepatitis, 12% regression
► histologic lesions:
   - fatty liver: macrovesicular steatosis alone
   - steatohepatitis: macrovesicular steatosis, cytologic ballooning, Mallory bodies, mixed, predominantly poly infiltration, perisinusoidal fibrosis
   - cirrhosis
► steroids helpful if Maddrey discriminant function [(DF) = 4.6[PT] + bili ÷ 17.1] is > 32; dose: prednisone 30–40 mg/day × 4 weeks with 2-week taper

TABLE 9-6
INDICATIONS AND RECOMMENDATIONS FOR ANTIVIRAL THERAPY OF CHRONIC HEPATITIS C

Standard indications for therapy

Elevated ALT activity
Fibrosis or moderate to severe hepatitis on liver biopsy
Detectable HCV RNA

Retreatment recommended

Relapsers after an initial course of interferon
    A 6-month course of combination interferon-ribavirin or a course of
        interferon monotherapy longer in duration than the original course

Antiviral therapy not recommended routinely but management decisions made on an individual basis

Children (age < 18 y)
Age > 60 y
Mild hepatitis on liver biopsy
Compensated cirrhosis
Patients with HIV infection and normal CD4 counts
Maintenance therapy in repeated relapsers
Nonresponders to a course of recombinant interferon—can be offered a
    48-wk course of consensus interferon, 15 μg three times a week (clin-
    ical trials underway to assess benefit of long-term "suppressive"
    therapy with other regimens)

Long-term therapy recommended

Cutaneous vasculitis and glomerulonephritis associated with chronic
    hepatitis C

Antiviral therapy not recommended

Decompensated cirrhosis
Normal ALT activity

Therapeutic regimens

First-line treatment: INF-α 3 million units subcutaneously three times a
    week plus ribavirin 1000 mg/d (weight < 75 kg) to 1200 mg/d
    (weight ≥ 75 kg) orally
    Duration of therapy: Genotype 1: 48 wks
                         Genotypes 2 and 3: 24 wks
Alternative regimen: INF-α monotherapy 3 million units (of recombinant
    interferon alfa-2a or alfa-2b or 9 μg of consensus interferon) subcuta-
    neously three times a week for 48 wks (primarily for patients in
    whom combination therapy is contraindicated or not tolerated)

Features associated with reduced responsiveness

Advanced histologic lesion (e.g., advanced cirrhosis)
Long-duration disease
Genotype 1
High-level HCV RNA (> 2 million copies/mL)
High HCV quasispecies diversity

TABLE 9-7
PATIENTS WITH CHRONIC HEPATITIS B WHO ARE CANDIDATES FOR ANTIVIRAL THERAPY

	Interferon	Lamivudine
Detectable markers of HBV replication	Yes	Yes
Elevated ALT activity	Yes	Yes
Chronic hepatitis on liver biopsy	Yes	Yes
Immunocompetence	Yes	Yes
Immunosuppression	No	Yes
Acquisition of infection in adulthood (Western)	Yes	Yes
Acquisition of infection in childhood (Asian)	No	Yes
Compensated liver disease	Yes	Yes
Decompensated liver disease	No	Yes
"Wild-type" chronic hepatitis B	Yes	Yes
Pre-core mutant hepatitis B	No	Yes
Prior nonresponse to interferon	No	Yes

TABLE 9-8
INDICATIONS FOR VACCINATION

Indications for HAV vaccination in adults	Indications for HBV vaccination in adults
Persons traveling to or working in countries with high or intermediate endemicity of infection	Health care workers
Men who have sex with men	Public safety workers with exposure to blood in the workplace
Illegal drug users (injection and noninjection)	Clients and staff of institutions for the developmentally disabled, day care centers, schools
Persons who have occupational risk for infection	Hemodialysis patients
Persons who have clotting factor disorders/receive clotting factor concentrates	Persons who have clotting factor disorders/receive clotting factor concentrates
Persons who have chronic liver disease	Household contacts and sex partners of HBV carriers
Persons who either are awaiting or have received liver transplantation	Adoptees from countries where HBV infection is endemic
Persons who work as food handlers in areas where such vaccination is cost-effective	International travelers who plan to spend more than 6 months in endemic area, who will have close contact with the local population, or who are likely to have contact with blood or sexual contact with residents
	Men who have sex with men
	HIV-infected persons
	Sexually active heterosexual men and women who recently acquired other sexually transmitted diseases, who are sex workers, or who have a history of sexual activity with more than one partner in the previous 6 months.
	Inmates of long-term correctional facilities

TABLE 9-9
INDICATIONS FOR LIVER TRANSPLANTATION IN FULMINANT (ACUTE) HEPATIC FAILURE (FHF)[a]

Patients with acetaminophen-induced FHF
  pH < 7.3 (irrespective of stage of encephalopathy)
  or
  PT > 100 s (INR > 6.5) and serum creatinine > 3.4 mg/dL in patients
    with stage III or IV encephalopathy
Other causes of FHF
  PT > 100 s (INR > 6.5) (irrespective of stage of encephalopathy)
or
Any three of the following:
  Age < 10 or > 40 y
  Any cause other than acetaminophen-induced disease or hepatitis
    A or B
  Duration of jaundice prior to onset of encephalopathy > 7 d
  PT > 50 s (INR > 3.5)
  Serum bilirubin > 17.5 mg/dL

[a]Adapted, with permission from O'Grady JG, et al. Early indicators of prognosis in fulminant hepatic failure. *Gastroenterology* 1989;97:439.
NOTE: PT, prothrombin time; INR, international normalized ratio.

REFERENCES

1. Everson GT, Trouillot TE. Current treatment strategies for hepatitis A, B, and C. *Gastroenterol Endoscop News* 2001;52(10):39–45.

2. Davis GL. Current treatment for chronic hepatitis C. *Rev Gastroenterol Dis* 2001;1(2):59–72.

3. Baker DE. Pegylated interferons. *Rev Gastroenterol Dis* 2001;1(2):87–99.

4. Baker DE. Pegylated interferon plus ribavirin for the treatment of chronic hepatitis C. *Rev Gastroenterol Dis* 2003;3(2):93–109.

5. Hefferman DJ, Terrault NA. Treatment of chronic hepatitis B virus infection. *Pract Gastroenterol* 2001;XXV(10):41–54.

6. Viernes ME, Byrne TJ, McHutchison JG. Current therapy of chronic hepatitis C infection. *Pract Gastroenterol* 2001; XXV(7):14–25.

7. Shaib YH, Vega KJ, Jamal MM. Approach to patients with hepatitis C and persistently normal alanine aminotransferase levels. *Clin Perspect Gastroenterol* 2000;3(5):252–258.

8. Komanduri S, Cotler SJ. Hepatitis C. *Clin Perspect Gastroenterol* 2002;5(2):91–99.

9. Pinto AG, Kwo PY. Pegylated interferon. *Clin Perspect Gastroenterol* 2002;5(5):292–296.

10. McNally PR. *GI/Liver Secrets.* 2nd ed. Philadelphia: Hanley & Belfus, 2001.

11. Emory TS, Carpenter HA, Gostout CJ, Sobin CJ. *Atlas of Gastrointestinal Endoscopy & Endoscopic Biopsies.* Washington DC: Armed Forces Institute of Pathology, 2000.

12. Bacon BR, DiBisceglie AM. *Liver Disease Diagnosis and Management.* Philadelphia: Churchill Livingstone, 2000.

13. Edwards ZC. Gastroenterology. In: Edwards TI, Mayer T, eds. *Urgent Care Medicine.* New York: McGraw-Hill, 2002:327.

14. Lauer GM, Walker BD. Hepatitis C virus infection. *N Engl J Med* 2001;345(1):41–48.

15. Howell C, Jeffers L, Hoofnagle JH. Hepatitis C in African Americans: summary of a workshop. *Gastroenterology* 2000;119:1385–1396.

16. Persico M, Persico E, Suozzo R, et al. Natural history of hepatitis C virus carriers with persistently elevated aminotransferase levels. *Gastroenterology* 2000;118:760–764.

17. Liang TJ, Rehermann B, Seeff LB, et al. Pathogenesis, natural history, treatment, and prevention of hepatitis C. *Ann Intern Med* 2000;132(4): 296–304.

18. Jaeckel E, Cornberg M, Wedemeyer H, et al. Treatment of acute hepatitis C with interferon alfa 2-b. *N Engl J Med* 2001;345(20):1452–1457.

19. Russo MW, Fried MW. Side effects of therapy for chronic hepatitis C. *Gastroenterology* 2003;124:1711–1719.

20. Herrine SK. Approach to the patient with chronic hepatitis C virus infection. *Ann Intern Med* 2002;136:747–757.

21. Yang HI, Lu SN, Liaw YF, et al. Hepatitis Be antigen and the risk of hepatocellular carcinoma. *N Engl J Med* 2002;347(3):168–174.

22. Sulkowski MS, Thomas DL. Hepatitis C in the HIV-infected person. *Ann Intern Med* 2003;138:197–207.

CHAPTER 10

AUTOIMMUNE LIVER DISEASE

AUTOIMMUNE LIVER DISEASE
Highlights

▶ **Helpful in differentiating syndromes:**
  • gender
  • symptoms and demographics
  • lab profile
▶ **Major Syndromes:**
  • autoimmune hepatitis
  • primary biliary cirrhosis
  • primary sclerosing cholangitis
  • overlap syndromes

Demographics

▶ **Autoimmune hepatitis** - female:male = 4–5:1; 10% of all cases of chronic hepatitis; bimodal age distribution - children and young adults (up to age 30) and 5th–6th decade; association with HLA-DR3, DR52, and DR4 antigens, C4a gene deletion seen in some young patients; fetal death in 15% of pregnancies and exacerbation of disease in 10–15% during pregnancy; non-responders - HLA-DR3

▶ **Primary biliary cirrhosis** - 50 cases/million; 95% female; mean age of 40–50; increased frequency of HLA-DRW8; 20% with other autoimmune disorders; slowly progressive with mean of 17 years to development of sx; 7 years avg time to death after development of sx; 50% 2-year survival once bili > 10

▶ **Primary sclerosing cholangitis** - 50 cases/million; 75% male; mean age of 40–50; 60–80% with HLA-B8 and/or HLA-DR3, also increased risk with HLA-DR3 and DRw52a; 75% with co-existent ulcerative colitis but no correlation between clinical course of PSC and IBD and total colectomy does not impact PSC; 50% of cases move from asxtic to sxtic over course of 5 years; single greatest risk factor for cholangiocarcinoma (1% per year ETOHA triples risk); increased risk of colon ca; median time from dx to end-stage liver dz of 12 years

▶ **Overlap syndromes** - sx similar to those in PBC, PSC, and autoimmune hepatitis; more common in female than male; mean age of 40–50; autoimmune cholangiopathy = AMA negative primary biliary cirrhosis

Symptoms/Signs/Labs

▶ **Autoimmune hepatitis** - predominant sx is fatigue, also anorexia, malaise, acute hepatitis (30%), acne, amenorrhea, arthralgias, autoimmune thyroid disease; majority with cirrhosis at time of dx; ALT and AST values in the 100's with ALT > AST, elevated TP and globulins; may get false-positive HIV and HCV; degree of elevation of ANA or anti-smooth muscle Ab not predictive of disease severity or prognosis; low albumin and increased PT predict development of cirrhosis; liver bx - portal mononuclear and plasma cell infiltrate (interface hepatitis/piecemeal necrosis), sparing of bile ducts, bridging fibrosis, cirrhosis, balloon degeneration

▶ **Primary biliary cirrhosis** - pruritus, jaundice: may subside spontaneously but becomes chronic and progressive with cirrhosis, xanthelasmas on eyelids, hands, and feet, osteoporosis with bone pain and fx, sicca syndrome in 50%, renal tubular acidosis in 50%, ? increased risk of breast ca, cirrhosis, increased risk of HCC; + anti-mitochondrial Ab (AMA - M2, M4, M8, M9 seen in PBC) diagnostic and seen in 95%, elevated alk phos, + ANA in 20%, steady rise of bili in cirrhosis, increased copper and urinary copper excretion, decreased albumin and increased PT with advanced disease, elevated cholesterol in 300–400 range but frequently involves HDL elevation; liver bx:

  • stage I: florid bile duct lesion with intense portal inflammation surrounding damaged duct
  • stage II: bile duct destruction and proliferation (biliary piecemeal)

- stage III: progressive bile duct loss with bridging fibrosis
- stage IV: cirrhosis, positive copper stain
- ▶ **Primary sclerosing cholangitis** - jaundice, cirrhosis, weight loss, fatigue; elevated alk phos, normal–elevated AST, ALT, elevated cholesterol, elevated serum and hepatic copper and ceruloplasmin; + ANA in 30%, + ANCA in 80%
- ▶ **Overlap syndromes** - elevated alk phos, normal bili, normal to elevated ALT and AST, + ANA, negative AMA and pANCA, + ASMA in 50%; liver bx - bile duct damage and proliferation, periportal granuloma, normal ERCP with no stricture formation in large bile ducts

Diagnosis

- ▶ **Autoimmune hepatitis:**
  - type I: + ANA, ASMA (anti-smooth muscle, anti-actin antibody)
  - type II: + anti-LKM1; type II more common in children
  - type III: + anti-soluble liver Ag
    - 1993 criteria:
      - LFT elevation > 6 months
      - 3–20-fold AST and ALT elevation
      - 1.5-fold elevation in serum gamma globulins
      - ANA > 1:40
      - ASMA > 1:80 or anti-LKM1 > 1:80
      - hepatitis due to Rx, virus, ETOH, hemochromatosis, Wilson disease, and 1 alpha antitrypsin deficiency ruled out
- ▶ **Primary biliary cirrhosis** - + AMA in 95%
- ▶ **Primary sclerosing cholangitis** - multifocal strictures and irregularity involving intrahepatic and/or bile ducts; ERCP - "chain of beads"; liver bx: onion-skin cholangitis
- ▶ **Overlap syndromes** - + antibody to carbonic anhydrase II

Treatment

- ▶ **Autoimmune hepatitis:**
  - initial: (a) prednisone at 20–30 mg; (b) prednisone at 10–20 mg + azathioprine at 50–100 mg

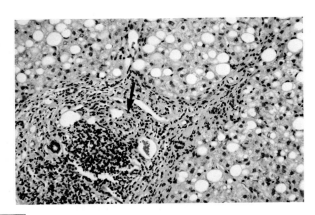

FIGURE 10-1
Immunoserologic markers of autoimmune hepatitis. (Reproduced with permission from Friedman SL, McQuaid KR, Grendell JH, *Current Diagnosis & Treatment in Gastroenterology*. Lange Medical Books/McGraw-Hill, 2003.)

- maintenance: (a) prednisone 5–15 mg or azathioprine at 2 mg/kg; (b) prednisone at 5–10 mg + azathioprine at 50–150 mg; treatment should be for 1–2 years, and reduction in ALT, AST, and globulin levels may take 1–3 months. Relapse occurs in 60% on withdrawal of tx, so long-term tx may be necessary.

TABLE 10-1
INDICATIONS FOR TREATMENT OF AUTOIMMUNE HEPATITIS

Absolute	Relative	None
Sustained serum AST level > 10-fold normal Sustained serum AST level > 5-fold normal and serum γ-globulin level more than twice normal Bridging necrosis Multilobular necrosis Incapacitating symptoms	Moderate serum AST and γ-globulin levels Interface hepatitis Moderate symptoms Disease progression	Mild or minimal serum AST and γ-globulin levels Cirrhosis with little or no inflammation Minimal or no symptoms Ascites, encephalopathy, or variceal bleeding and little or no inflammatory activity

TABLE 10-2
TREATMENT REGIMENS FOR AUTOIMMUNE HEPATITIS

Prednisone (daily dose)	Combination therapy (daily dose)	
	Prednisone	Azathioprine
60 mg for 1 wk 40 mg for 1 wk 30 mg for 2 wks 20 mg until end point	30 mg for 1 wk 20 mg for 1 wk 15 mg for 2 wks 10 mg until end point	50 mg until end point
Relative contraindications		
Postmenopausal Osteopenia Emotional lability Acne or cushingoid features Obesity Labile hypertension Brittle diabetes	Cytopenia Active neoplasm Pregnancy or desire for pregnancy Azothioprine intolerance Low thiopurine methyltransferase activity Short (≤ 6 mos) treatment trial	

- liver transplantation: recurrence of disease in 15–40%; 92% 5-year survival
▶ **Primary biliary cirrhosis:**
  1. *General:*
     a. pruritus - antihistamine, cholestyramine, rifampin, UDCA (slows progression to fibrosis and decreases LFTs but does not decrease time to transplant or increase survival; dose at 10–15 mg/kg/day)
     b. osteoporosis - calcium at 1300 mg/day + vit D at 5000 U/day
     c. vitamin malabsorption - supplementation of vits D, A, E, K
     d. hypercholesterolemia - Rx only if high LDL or VLDL
  2. *Liver transplantation, indicated if:* bili ≥ 2–10, severe osteoporosis with vertebral fx or collapse, intractable pruritus, albumin < 3, end-stage liver disease; 90–95% 2-year survival
▶ **Primary sclerosing cholangitis:**
  1. Stenting of high-grade strictures with major ducts in patients with jaundice
  2. Liver transplantation treatment of choice - indicated in prolonged jaundice, recurrent episodes of biliary sepsis, domi-

nant stricture suggestive of cholangiocarcinoma (found in 15% at time of surgery), intractable pruritus, end-stage liver disease

3. UDCA - improves LFTs and reduces risk of colonic dysplasia in patients with UC by 80%; does not reduce time to ESLD or transplant

▶ **Overlap syndromes** - dependent on sx-predominant syndrome, so may include UDCA, steroids, liver transplantation

TABLE 10-3
AUTOIMMUNE LIVER DISEASE

	PBC	PSC	Autoimmune overlap syndrome
Frequency	50 cases/million	50 cases/million	
Gender distribution	Female:male = 9:1	Male:female = 2:1	
Mean age	20 – 40 y	20 – 50 y	
Bile duct status	Small duct dz	Large duct dz	
Co-existent disease	Autoimmune—sicca 50%, RA* 20%, hypothyroidism 20%, scleroderma and Sjögren's 10%	IBD—UC 80%, Crohn's 5%, scleroderma and mixed connective tissue disease 10%	
Liver biopsy	Diagnostic	Nonspecific	Features consistent with PBC or autoimmune hepatitis
ERCP	Normal	Diagnostic	Normal
Alk phos, copper	Elevated	Elevated	Elevated
ALT, bili	Normal–elevated	Normal–elevated	Usually normal
Cholesterol	Elevated	Normal–elevated	
ANA +	20%	33%	✓
ASMA +	20%	65%	50%
AMA +	95%	0%	—
ANCA +		85%	✓
Carbonic anhydrase II	—	—	
HLA status	DRW8	B8, DR3	

*RA, rheumatoid arthritis.

REFERENCES

1. Bacon BR, DiBisceglie AM. *Liver Disease Diagnosis and Management*. Philadelphia: Churchill Livingstone, 2000.
2. Feldman M, Scharschmidt BF, Sleisenger MH. *Sleisenger & Fordtran's Gastrointestinal and Liver Disease*. 6th ed. Philadelphia: WB Saunders, 1998.
3. Yamada Y, ed. *Textbook of Gastroenterology*. 3rd ed. Philadelphia: Lippincott Williams & Wilkins, 1999.
4. Goldman L, Bennett JC, Eds. *Cecil Textbook of Medicine*. 21st ed. Philadelphia: WB Saunders, 2000.

CHAPTER 11

THE PORPHYRIAS

PORPHYRIAS
Highlights

▶ **Helpful in differentiating syndromes:**
  - gender
  - symptoms and demographics
  - lab profile
▶ **Major Syndromes:**
  - 5 *hepatic* porphyrias:
    1. acute intermittent porphyria (AIP)
    2. ALA (δ-aminolevulinic acid) dehydrase deficiency
    3. hereditary coproporphyria (HCP)
    4. variegate porphyria
    5. porphyria cutanea tarda (PCT)
  - 4 *erythropoietic* porphyrias:
    1. protoporphyria
    2. congenital erythropoietic porphyria
    3. erythropoietic coproporphyria
    4. hepatoerythropoietic porphyria
▶ All of the hepatic porphyrias except porphyria cutanea tarda are associated with acute neurologic crises.
▶ Lead toxicity may mimic acute hepatic porphyria.
▶ Acute attacks are more common in women, usually after onset of puberty, and often associated with the luteal phase of menstruation.

TABLE 11-1
DEMOGRAPHICS/SYMPTOMS—SIGNS—LABS/DIAGNOSIS/TREATMENT

Disease	Features	Diagnosis	Treatment
Porphyrias		Detection of excess PBG or porphyrins in urine, blood, or stool; fluorescence of liver and stool	
Acute attacks			- pain control with narcotics prn - control of hypertension and tachycardia with β-blocker - glucose/carbohydrate therapy ≥300 g/d glucose - IV hematin, 3–4 mg/kg × 3–5 d - LHRH[b] analog for female with luteal phase recurrence - monitor for neuromuscular/respiratory dysfunction - remove exacerbating drugs/chemicals
Chronic or recurrent disease			*General:* - avoid ETOH, exacerbating Rx/chemicals - wear sunscreen and opaque clothing - treat skin infection promptly - avoid severe dieting or low protein & carbohydrate intake - test 1st degree relatives *PCT:[c]* - phlebotomy

	- treat hepatitis C if present - use chloroquine, hydroxychloro-quine, or alkalization of urine to ↑ urinary porphyrin excretion *Protoporphyria:* - oral β-carotene - RBC transfusion, iron - cholestyramine, activated charcoal - liver transplantation
ALA^d dehydrase deficiency	- decreased conversion of ALA to por-phobilinogen - autosomal recessive - sx: recurrent, severe neurologic attacks with marked abd pain and respiratory and bulbar paralysis possible
Acute intermit-tent porphyria	- most common porphyria in U.S. - autosomal dominant - defective gene on chromosome 11q24 and carried by 5–10/100,000 - deficiency of PBG deaminase - female presentation in 3rd decade male presentation in 4th decade - attacks precipitated by Rx

continued

TABLE 11-1
DEMOGRAPHICS/SYMPTOMS–SIGNS–LABS/DIAGNOSIS/TREATMENT (CONTINUED)

Disease	Features	Diagnosis	Treatment
	- sx: colicky abd pain frequently accompanied by constipation, N&V; also, trunk and extremity paresthesias, motor neuropathy, tachycardia, hypertension, areflexia, bulbar findings, depression, rage, anxiety, frank psychosis and delirium, hyponatremia (→ risk of seizure or coma), death possible as result of infection associated with recurrent aspiration or pulmonary paralysis		
Hereditary coproporphyria	- deficiency of coproporphyrinogen oxidase → ↑ coproporphyrin III - autosomal dominant - defect on gene 9 - sx: similar to AIP[e], also vesiculobullous dermatitis of face, hands, other exposed skin		
Variegate porphyria	- deficiency of protoporphyrinogen oxidase - autosomal dominant - defective gene on chromosome 1q22 - increased incidence in S. Africa - sx: variable, may see episodes similar to AIP, photosensitivity as in HCP,[f] or asymptomatic		

| Porphyria cutanea tarda | - deficiency of uroporphyrinogen decarboxylase
- autosomal dominant or sporadic
- 3 types with type I seen in 75%
- defective gene on chromosome 1q
- sx: photosensitivity + hepatic disease; ↑ AST, ALT, glucose intolerance
- association with hepatitis C (60 – 90% of PCT patients positive for hep C), iron overload |
| Erythropoietic porphyria | - deficiency in ferrochelatase
- defective gene on chromosome 18q22
- autosomal recessive or dominant
- sx: skin photosensitivity acutely manifest as stinging/burning/itching followed by erythema, edema, and scarring hypertrophic changes, mild anemia – hemolysis, pigmented gallstones |

[a]PBG, porphobilinogen; [b]LHRH, luteinizing hormone-releasing hormone; [c]PCT, porphyria cutanea tarda; [d]δ-aminolevulinic acid; [e]AIP, acute intermittent porphyria; [f]HCP, hereditary coproporphyria.

TABLE 11-2
CLASSIFICATION OF THE PORPHYRIAS

Type	Enzyme defect	Inheritance	Clinical type
Hepatic porphyria			
Acute intermittent porphyria	PBG[a] deaminase	Dominant	Acute, neurologic
Hereditary coproporphyria	COPROgen[b] oxidase	Dominant	Acute, neurologic (+ cutaneous)
Variegate porphyria	PROTOgen[c] oxidase	Dominant	Acute, neurologic (+ cutaneous)
δ-ALAuria[f]	PBG synthase	Recessive	Acute, neurologic
Cutanea tarda	UROgen[e] decarboxylase	Dominant (+ acquired?)	Chronic, cutaneous
Lead intoxication	PBG synthase + COPRO oxidase	(Acquired)	Neurologic
"Toxic" porphyria	UROgen decarboxylase	(Acquired)	Cutaneous
Erythropoietic porphyria			
Congenital erythropoietic porphyria	UROgen synthase	Recessive	Cutaneous
Protoporphyria	Heme synthase	Dominant	Cutaneous (+ hepatic)

[a]PBG, porphobilinogen; [b]COPROgen, coproporphyrinogen; [c]PROTOgen, protoporphyrinogen; [d]UROgen, uroporphyrinogen; [e]δ-ALA, δ-aminolevulinic acid.

TABLE 11-3
UNSAFE AND SAFE DRUGS IN PORPHYRIA[a]

	Unsafe	Believed to be safe
Anticonvulsants	**Barbiturates**	Bromides
	Carbamazepine	Diazepam
	Clonazepam	Magnesium sulfate
	Ethosuximide	
	Hydantoins	
	Phenytoin	
	Primidone	
	Valproic acid	
Hypnotics or	**Barbiturates**	Chloral hydrate
sedatives	Chlordiazepoxide	Chlorpromazine
	Ethchlorvynol	Diphenhydramine
	Glutethimide	Lithium
	Meprobamate	Lorazepam
	Methyprylon	Meclizine
		Trifluoperazine
Other drugs	α-**Methyldopa**	ACTH
	Danazol	Allopurinol
	Diclofenac	Aminoglycosides
	Ergot preparations	Aspirin
	Estrogens	Atropine
	Griseofulvin	Codeine
	Imipramine	Colchicine
	Pentazocine	Dexamethasone
	Pyrazinamide	Furosemide
	Sulfonamides	Ibuprofen
	Sulfonylureas	Insulin
		Meperidine
		Morphine
		Naproxen
		Penicillins
		Warfarin

[a]The agents in **bold print** have been implicated repeatedly in acute attacks. For the other "unsafe" compounds, the clinical information is anecdotal but supported by tests in experimental animals or *in vitro*.

REFERENCES

1. Bacon BR, DiBisceglie AM. *Liver Disease Diagnosis and Management.* Philadelphia: Churchill Livingstone, 2000.
2. Feldman M, Scharschmidt BF, Sleisenger MH. *Sleisenger & Fordtran's Gastrointestinal and Liver Disease.* 6th ed. Philadelphia: WB Saunders, 1998.
3. Yamada Y, ed. *Textbook of Gastroenterology.* 3rd ed. Philadelphia: Lippincott Williams & Wilkins, 1999.
4. Goldman L, Bennett JC, eds. *Cecil Textbook of Medicine.* 21st ed. Philadelphia: WB Saunders, 2000.

CHAPTER 12

HEPATOLOGY DRUG REVIEW

HEPATOLOGY DRUG REVIEW
General Information

▶ Most common drug reaction of all drugs is cholestasis.

▶ Most common histologic pattern of drug injury is nonspecific hepatitis.

▶ Metabolite rather than native drug is usually offending agent.

▶ risk factors for drug-induced hepatotoxicity - age > 50, female gender, obesity, ETOH use, previous history of drug-induced hepatotoxicity, polypharmacy

▶ subclinical liver injury - elevated AST/ALT/alk phos, occurs in 5–50% of patients, lab elevations usually < 3 × normal, lab elevations may resolve spontaneously, Rx may be continued if LFTs monitored and stable over time; discontinue drug if LFTs continue to rise or are > 2.5 × normal range

▶ risk factors for drug-induced hepatotoxicity - age > 50, female gender, obesity, ETOH use, previous history of drug-induced hepatotoxicity, polypharmacy

TABLE 12-1
HIGHLIGHTS OF HEPATIC DRUG REACTIONS

Feature	Intrinsic	Idiosyncratic
Dose-dependent	✓	
Predictable	✓	
Genetic		✓
Type	Hepatocellular damage; hepatitis	Cell-mediated; cholestasis
Cause	Metabolic	Hypersensitivity
Drugs	Acetaminophen, INH, chloroform, Amanita mushrooms	NSAID, oral hypoglycemics, Dilantin, TMP-SMX, H2 blockers, salicylate

TABLE 12-2
SIGNS OF HEPATIC DRUG REACTIONS

Type	Exposure	Clinical	Recurrence
Hypersensitivity	Weeks	Rash, fever, EOS, Stevens-Johnson	Prompt
Aberrant metabolism	Months	Liver only	Delayed
Mixed	Variable	Both	Prompt

Specific Risk-Factor Associations

► age > 35 - INH
► geriatric - INH, methotrexate, NSAIDs, PCN
► pediatric age - salicylate, erythro, valproate
► female - INH, diclofenac, sulindac, PCN
► male - azathioprine
► obesity - inhaled anesthetics, methotrexate
► ETOH - acetaminophen, inhaled anesthetics, INH, cocaine, vit A, methotrexate
► cirrhosis - methotrexate, oncologic agents
► polypharmacy with hepatic cytochrome inducers - Dilantin, phenobarbital, rifampin, ETOH
► increase cyclosporine levels - erythro, ketoconazole, cimetidine
► acetaminophen toxicity - ETOH, anti-sz Rx, rifampin
► slow acetylator - INH, sulfonamides, dihydralazine
► African or Asian - INH

TABLE 12-3
DRUGS COMMONLY ASSOCIATED WITH LIVER ABNORMALITIES USED IN THE TREATMENT
OF HIV AND ITS COMPLICATIONS

Predominantly hepatocellular disease	Predominantly cholestatic disease
Clarithromycin	Rifampin
Delaviridine	Ketoconazole
Didanosine (ddl)	TMP-SMX
Dideoxycytidine (ddC)	Dapsone
Efavirenz	
Indinavir	
Isoniazid	
Ketoconazole	
Nelfinavir	
Nevirapine	
Pentamidine	
Ritonavir	
Saquinavir	
Stavudine (d4T)	
TMP-SMX	
Zidovudine	

▶ pre-existing liver disease - INH, methotrexate
▶ AIDS - PCN, sulfonamides (Table 12–3)
▶ renal insufficiency - allopurinol, methotrexate
▶ JRA, Still's disease - ASA

Morphologic Changes

▶ Necrosis - INH, methyldopa, acetaminophen, halothane
▶ autoimmune hepatitis - nitrofurantoin, diclofenac, methyldopa, INH, amiodarone, minocycline, clometacine (NSAIDs)
▶ granulomatous hepatitis - quinidine, allopurinol, sulfonylureas
▶ cholestasis - NSAIDs, H2 blockers, testosterone, estrogen, progesterone, BCP, erythro, haloperidol, captopril, TMP-SMX
▶ fibrosis - methotrexate, vit A
▶ steatosis:
  1. macrovesicular - glucocorticoids, methotrexate, amiodarone, estrogen
  2. microvesicular - TCN, valproate, salicylate, zidovudine, NSAIDs: piroxicam, naproxen, ibuprofen, ketoprofen,
▶ phospholipidosis - amiodarone, sulfonamides, tamoxifen, griseofulvin

TABLE 12-4
PRINCIPAL ALTERATIONS OF HEPATIC MORPHOLOGY PRODUCED BY SOME COMMONLY
USED DRUGS AND CHEMICALS[a]

Principal morphologic change	Class of agent	Example
Cholestasis	Anabolic steroid	Methyl testosterone
	Antiinflammatory	Sulindac
	Antithyroid	Methimazole
	Antibiotic	Erythromycin estolate, nitrofurantoin, rifampin, amoxicillin-clavulinic acid, oxacillin
	Oral contraceptive	Norethynodrel with mestranol
	Oral hypoglycemic	Chlorpropamide
	Tranquilizer	Chlorpromazine[b]
	Oncotherapeutic	Anabolic steroids, busulfan, tamoxifen
	Immunosuppressive	Cyclosporine
	Anticonvulsant	Carbamazine
	Calcium channel blocker	Nifedipine, verapamil
Fatty liver	Antibiotic	Tetracycline
	Anticonvulsant	Sodium valproate
	Antiarrhythmic	Amiodarone
	Antiviral	Dideoxynucleosides (e.g., zidovudine) protease inhibitors (e.g., indinavir, ritonavir)
	Oncotherapeutic	Asparaginase, methotrexate
Hepatitis	Anesthetic	Halothane[c]
	Anticonvulsant	Phenytoin, carbamazine
	Antihypertensive	Methyldopa,[c] captopril, enalapril
	Antibiotic	Isoniazid,[c] rifampin, nitrofurantoin
	Diuretic	Chlorothiazide
	Laxative	Oxyphenisatin[c]
	Antidepressant	Iproniazid, amitriptyline, imipramine
	Antiinflammatory	Ibuprofen, indomethacin, diclofenac, sulindac
	Antifungal	Ketoconazole, fluconazole, itraconazole
	Antiviral	Zidovudine, dideoxy inosine
	Calcium channel blocker	Nifedipine, verapamil, diltiazem
	Antiandrogen	Flutamide

continued

TABLE 12-4
PRINCIPAL ALTERATIONS OF HEPATIC MORPHOLOGY PRODUCED BY SOME COMMONLY
USED DRUGS AND CHEMICALS[a] (CONTINUED)

Principal morphologic change	Class of agent	Example
Mixed hepatitis/cholestatic	Immunosuppressive	Azathioprine
	Lipid-lowering	Nicotinic acid, lovastatin
Toxic (necrosis)	Hydrocarbon	Carbon tetrachloride
	Metal	Yellow phosphorus
	Mushroom	Amanita phalloides
	Analgesic	Acetaminophen
	Solvent	Dimethylformamide
Granulomas	Antiinflammatory	Phenylbutazone
	Antibiotic	Sulfonamides
	Xanthine oxidase inhibitor	Allopurinol
	Antiarrhythmic	Quinidine
	Anticonvulsant	Carbamazine

[a]Several agents cause more than one type of liver lesion and appear under more than one category.
[b]Rarely associated with primary biliary cirrhosis-like lesion.
[c]Occasionally associated with chronic hepatitis or bridging hepatic necrosis or cirrhosis.

► vascular lesions - hepatic vein thrombosis: BCP; veno-occlusive dz: alkaloids, BMT, chemo, XRT; peliosis hepatis: anabolic steroids, tamoxifen, azathioprine
► neoplastic lesions:
  1. adenoma - BCP
  2. HCC - aflatoxin
  3. angiosarcoma - vinyl chloride, anabolic steroids, nitrosamines

Drug-Specific Highlights

► isoniazid:
  • ↑ LFTs in 20% and usually seen within 2 months of starting therapy
  • LFT elevation usually resolves spontaneously
  • severe injury in 1% (2% for those whose age is > 50), fulminant in 10%
  • increased risk if female gender

▶ acetaminophen:
  - average dose in overdose: 10–15 g in suicide attempts
  - usually result of therapeutic "misadventure" involving ETOH (2 drinks/day enough to create a px)
  - ↑ AST, ALT with levels which may be > 15,000
  - tx: gastric lavage + N-acetylcysteine (effective even up to 24 hours following overdose)
  - indications for liver transplantation: pH < 7.3, PT > 100, creat > 3, stage 3–4 encephalopathy
▶ amoxicillin - loss of bile ducts
▶ Dilantin - effect usually seen within first 3 weeks

Miscellaneous

▶ induce hepatic cytochromes - ETOH, phenytoin, phenobarbital, rifampin, isoniazid, glucocorticoids, omeprazole
▶ ↑ cyclosporine levels - erythromycin, ketoconazole, cimetidine
▶ intrinsic toxicity - ↑ AST, ALT

REFERENCES

1. Hardman JG, Limbird LE, Gilman AG, eds. *Goodman & Gilman's: The Pharmacologic Basis of Therapeutics.* 10th ed. New York: McGraw-Hill, 2001.
2. Friedman SL, McQuaid KR, Grendell JH. *Diagnosis & Treatment in Gastroenterology.* New York: Lange Medical Books/McGraw-Hill, 2003.
3. Feldman M, Scharschmidt BF, Sleisenger MH. *Sleisenger & Fordtran's Gastrointestinal and Liver Disease.* 6th ed. Philadelphia: WB Saunders, 1998.
4. Yamada Y, ed. *Textbook of Gastroenterology.* 3rd ed. Philadelphia: Lippincott Williams & Wilkins, 1999.
5. Dharmarajan TS, Pitchumoni CS, Kumar KS. Drug-induced liver disease in older adults. *Pract Gastroenterol* 2001;XXV(3):43–60.
6. Lewis JH, guest editor. Drug-induced liver disease. In: *Gastroenterology Clinics of North America.* Philadelphia: WB Saunders, December 1995.
7. Braunwald E, Fauci AS, Kasper DL, et al. *Harrison's Principles of Internal Medicine.* 15th ed. New York: McGraw-Hill, 2001.

CHAPTER 13

GENETIC LIVER DISEASE

GENETIC LIVER DISEASE
Highlights

► **Helpful in differentiating syndromes:**
  • genetic profile
  • symptoms and demographics
  • lab profile
► **Major Syndromes:**
  • hemochromatosis
  • Wilson's disease
  • alpha-1 antitrypsin deficiency

Demographics

► **Hemochromatosis** - autosomal recessive, HLA-A haplotype, problem on chromosome 6: HFE gene - C282Y mutation (cysteine to tyrosine substitution at AA282) and/or H63D mutation (histidine to aspartate at AA63); hereditary hemochromatosis - usually homozygous for C282Y or heterozygous for C282Y and H63D;1:200–1:500 white population, most common in those of northern European descent; 30% of females and 10% of males who are homozygotes do not have Fe overload; diagnosis and treatment prior to development of cirrhosis results in normal life expectancy.

► **Wilson's disease** - autosomal recessive, male = female, 1 in 30,000; chromosome 13q14.3, involves up to 60 different mutations

► **alpha-1 antitrypsin deficiency** - most common genetic liver disease in infants and children; 1 in 1600 – 1 in 2800 live births; Z variant - PiZZ most common phenotype associated with liver dz and has 10–20% risk of liver dz; high risk of HCC in cirrhotics; 30% of cases have liver dz without lung dz

Symptoms/Signs/Labs

▶ **Hemochromatosis** - hepatomegaly, elevated LFTs, fatigue, abdominal pain, bronzing of skin, arthralgias, impotence, diabetes, cirrhosis, cardiomyopathy; 200× increased risk of HCC in cirrhotics; increased mortality secondary to HCC, diabetes, cardiomyopathy; liver bx - increased stainable iron in hepatocytes and bile duct cells with paucity in Kupffer cells

▶ **Wilson's disease** - most present with hepatic and/or neuro sx, with presentation before age 5 or after age 40 rare, avg age for hepatic sx 10–14 yo and neuro 19–22 yo, chronic hepatitis, fibrosis, cirrhosis, fulminant hepatic failure, neuropsychiatric manifestations (depression, mood disorders, personality changes), Kayser-Fleischer rings, decreased alk phos, decreased uric acid, Coombs negative hemolytic anemia, tremor, hypertonicity, choreoathetosis, parkinsonian-like features, splenomegaly, osteopenia, distal RTA, hypercalciuria, polyarthritis, CHF, arrhythmia, glucose intolerance, amenorrhea; liver presentations: (1) fulminant hepatic failure, (2) chronic hepatitis, (3) cirrhosis; liver bx - fatty infiltration, cirrhosis

▶ **alpha-1 antitrypsin deficiency** - neonatal hepatitis, precocious emphysema, abdominal pain, hepatomegaly, variceal hemorrhage; liver bx - PAS-positive diastase resistant globules

Diagnosis

▶ **Hemochromatosis** - elevated iron (> 175), total iron binding capacity (TIBC) (< 300), ferritin (> 200 ng/mL in female, >300 in male), transferrin-iron saturation (TS: serum iron ÷ TIBC) > 45%; liver bx - > 4000 μg/g dry weight and hepatic iron index = 1.9 (hepatic iron index helps to distinguish between a heterozygote or alcoholic with Fe overload from a homozygote)

▶ **Wilson's disease** - low serum ceruloplasmin (< 20 mg/dL), slit-lamp exam, liver bx - hepatic copper > 250 μg/g dry weight (normal < 35), urinary copper > 100 μg/24 hours (normal < 30 μg/24 hours), serum copper < 80; genetic screening

TABLE 13-1
INTERPRETATION OF GENETIC TESTING FOR HEMOCHROMATOSIS

C282Y homozygote
This is the classic genetic pattern that is seen in > 90% of typical cases. Expression of disease ranges from no evidence of iron overload to massive iron overload with organ dysfunction. Siblings have approximately a one in four chance of being affected and should have genetic testing. For children to be affected, the other parent must be at least a heterozygote. If iron studies are normal, false-positive genetic testing or a nonexpressing homozygote should be considered.

C282Y/H63D - Compound heterozygote
This patient carries one copy of the major mutation and one copy of the minor mutation. Most patients with this genetic pattern have normal iron studies. A small percentage of compound heterozygotes have been found to have mild to moderate iron overload. Severe iron overload is usually seen in the setting of another concomitant risk factor (alcoholism, viral hepatitis).

C282Y heterozygote
This patient carries one copy of the major mutation. This pattern is seen in about 10% of the white population and is usually associated with normal iron studies. In rare cases, the iron studies are high in the range expected in a homozygote rather than a heterozygote. These cases may carry an unknown hemochromatosis mutation and liver biopsy is helpful to determine the need for venesection therapy.

H63D homozygote
This patient carries two copies of the minor mutation. Most patients with this genetic pattern have normal iron studies. A small percentage of these cases have been found to have mild to moderate iron overload. Severe iron overload is usually seen in the setting of another concomitant risk factor (alcoholism, viral hepatitis).

H63D heterozygote
This patient carries one copy of the minor mutation. This pattern is seen in about 20% of the white population and is usually associated with normal iron studies. This pattern is so common in the general population that the presence of iron overload may be related to another risk factor. Liver biopsy may be required to determine the cause of the iron overload and the need for treatment in these cases.

No HFE mutations
Iron overload has been described in families with mutations in other iron-related genes (transferrin receptor 2 and IREG1). Other hemochromatosis mutations will likely be discovered in the future. If iron overload is present without any HFE mutations, a careful history for other risk factors must be reviewed and liver biopsy may be useful to determine the cause of the iron overload and the need for treatment. Most of these are isolated, nonfamilial cases.

TABLE 13-2
TREATMENT OF WILSON'S DISEASE

Medication	Dosage	Comment
D-Penicillamine	25–30 mg/kg in divided doses,[a] 15 mg/kg for maintenance therapy	Initial therapy with lower dosage increased to full dosage over 1–2 wks time; monitoring for side effects is essential; dosage reduction for surgery and pregnancy necessary
Trientine	~20 mg/kg in divided doses,[a] 15 mg/kg for maintenance therapy	Initial therapy with lower dosage increased to full dosage over 1–2 wks time; initial hypersensitivity is rare, however, a reversible sideroblastic anemia may occur with long-term use; dosage reduction for surgery and pregnancy necessary
Zinc salts	25 mg bid or tid for pediatric patients, 50 mg tid for adults	Used as maintenance therapy or for initial therapy for asymptomatic patients, may be used adjunctively with chelating agent as initial therapy

[a]Rounded to the nearest 250 mg as these medications are supplied in 250-mg capsules.

appropriate in the following circumstances: (1) children with liver and/or neuro dz, (2) Fanconi syndrome, (3) decreased uric acid, (4) Kayser-Fleischer rings, (5) sibling with dz

▶ **alpha-1 antitrypsin deficiency** - phenotyping: most with chronic liver dz are homozygous for Z allele (PiZZ) or compound heterozygous for SZ (PiSZ); alpha-1 antitrypsin levels 10–15% of normal

Treatment

▶ **Hemochromatosis:**

1. phlebotomy - 500 mL weekly until mild anemia (Hct ≤ 75% of baseline) and ferritin < 50 ng/mL (may take up to 2 years). Phlebotomy may result in improvement in fatigue, LFT elevation, hepatomegaly, cardiac function, complications of portal hypertension but does not impact joint symptoms. Vit C should be avoided, as it increases iron absorption.

2. liver transplantation - 1-year and 5-year survivals of 60% and 40%, respectively, with decreased survival due to infection and cardiac complications

▶ **Wilson's disease:**

1. removal - penicillamine (1–2 g/day in 4 doses 30 minutes ac) or trientine (second- line tx, less potent and fewer side effects than penicillamine); need pyridoxine supplement as penicillamine tx depletes stores; may take weeks to months before response to tx; penicillamine may worsen neuro-psych sx; neuropsych sx less responsive than liver disease; side effects - rash, nephrotic syndrome, hypersensitivity disorder; maintenance - zinc at 150 mg/day in 3 doses + low copper diet (avoid shellfish, chocolate, nuts, liver); urine excretion of 250–500 µg/day implies copper-depleted state.

2. liver transplantation - curative

▶ **alpha-1 antitrypsin deficiency** - liver transplantation 65% long-term survival rate

REFERENCES

1. Bowlus CL. Genetic testing in hemochromatosis. *Pract Gastroenterol* 2001;XXV(9): 44–56.
2. Schilsky ML. Wilson's disease. *Clin Perspect Gastroenterol* 2002;5(4):234–243.
3. Bacon BR, DiBisceglie AM. *Liver Disease Diagnosis and Management*. Philadelphia: Churchill Livingstone, 2000.
4. Maddrey WC. Update in hepatology. *Ann Intern Med* 2001;134(3):216–223.
5. El-Serag HB, Inadom JM, Kowdley KV. Screening for hereditary hemochromatosis in siblings and children of affected patients. *Ann Intern Med* 2000;132:261–269.

CHAPTER 14

SURGICAL CONSIDERATIONS

LIVER

Highlights

- ▶ makes up to 5% of total body weight
- ▶ consumes 25% of total body oxygen
- ▶ dual blood supply from the portal vein (75%) and the hepatic artery (25%)
- ▶ produces up to 1 L of bile per day
- ▶ synthesizes albumin, fibrinogen, and prothrombin
- ▶ responsible for glycogenesis, glycogen storage, glycogenolysis, and the conversion of galactose to glucose
- ▶ **Major Syndromes:**
  - benign noncystic liver lesions
    - a. hemangioma
    - b. focal nodular hyperplasia
    - c. hepatic adenoma
  - liver cysts
    - a. polycystic disease
    - b. cystadenoma
    - c. hydatid liver cyst
  - hepatocellular carcinoma
  - hepatic abscess
    - a. pyogenic
    - b. amebic

Demographics

- ▶ **Benign noncystic liver lesions:**
  1. *Hemangioma* - most common nodule in liver; usually small but can be large, multiple lesions (may replace most of the

liver); rupture is rare; may cause congestive heart failure due to the formation of arteriovenous shunts and a consumptive coagulopathy; affects females 5× more than males

2. *Focal nodular hyperplasia (FNH)* - primarily affects women of reproductive age; has been linked to oral contraceptives; usually solitary lesion; does not rupture, hemorrhage, or undergo malignant change; characteristic central stellate scar

3. *Hepatic adenoma* - 90% found in 30–50 yo women; linked to oral contraceptives; usually solitary lesions; may rupture or hemorrhage; malignant change is possible

► **Liver cysts:**

1. *Polycystic disease* - autosomal recessive variant presents in childhood; autosomal dominant variant presents in adulthood; childhood form associated with polycystic renal disease and progressive renal insufficiency; adult variant is associated with cysts in the kidney, pancreas, spleen, ovaries, and lungs; in both variants liver failure is uncommon

2. *Cystadenoma* - 80% are middle-aged women; usually large; usually located in the right lobe; multilocular and contain clear mucinous material

3. *Hydatid liver cyst* - caused by the larval form of *Echinococcus granulosus*; *E. granulosus* requires two hosts: the primary host (canines) harbors the adult worm and an intermediate host (usually sheep, cattle, goats, deer, and caribou) harbors the larvae; humans are an accidental intermediate host following ingestion of unwashed vegetables contaminated with eggs; endemic to Italy, Greece, Bulgaria, Lebanon, Turkey, North Africa, Brazil, Uruguay, Argentina, Chile, and Peru

► **Hepatocellular carcinoma (HCC)** - most common solid tumor of the GI tract worldwide; associated with HBV and HBC; other risk factors include alcoholic cirrhosis, hemochromatosis, $\alpha1$ antitrypsin deficiency, Wilson's disease, tyrosinemia, and glycogen storage disease; rarely occurs in healthy livers

► **Hepatic abscess**

1. *Pyogenic* - most common abscess in the U.S.; usually gramnegative bacteria; highest incidence in 6th or 7th decade; usually seen in the right lobe; sources of infection include the biliary tract, pyelophlebitis, systemic bacteremia, cryptogenic, malignancy, and trauma

2. *Amebic* - caused by *Entamoeba histolytica*; common in tropical and subtropical climates worldwide; becoming more prevalent in the southwestern U.S.; infection occurs via a fecal-oral route with ingestion of the cyst form; cysts mature into an invasive trophozoite and travel to the liver; patients tend to be young men who are immigrants or who have recently traveled to endemic regions; Mexican immigrants are the predominant group seen in the U.S. with this disorder.

Symptoms/Signs/Labs

▶ **Benign noncystic liver lesions**
   1. *Hemangioma* - pain is associated with enlargement, otherwise, asymptomatic
   2. *Focal nodular hyperplasia (FNH)* - asymptomatic
   3. *Hepatic adenoma* - abd pain or noticeable mass; with rupture into the peritoneal space, patients may develop profuse bleeding and shock

▶ **Liver cysts**
   1. *Polycystic disease* - childhood variant is asymptomatic; adult variant may be asymptomatic or present as a complaint of upper abd fullness, mild pain, early satiety
   2. *Cyst adenoma* - asymptomatic
   3. *Hydatid liver cysts* - usually asymptomatic until they reach a large size; may have localized pain; liver may become adherent to the diaphragm or abd wall; may erode into the bile ducts and become infected (cyst will then present as an abscess); may erode into the bile ducts and produce transient obstructive jaundice and fever; rupture of cyst contents may produce an allergic reaction ranging from mild to severe anaphylaxis.

▶ **Hepatocellular carcinoma** - usually asymptomatic until dz is in its advanced stages; symptoms are usually abd pain, distention, weight loss, and new onset of bleeding, ascites, or jaundice; hepatomegaly, arterial bruit, spider angiomas, and evidence of portal hypertension may be appreciated on physical exam

▶ **Hepatic abscess** - pyogenic and amebic abscesses present very similarly; symptoms present in < 2 weeks; symptoms include fever, chills, malaise, anorexia, weight loss, pain, nausea, history of fever of unknown origin, and a long-standing respiratory infection before the onset of abd symptoms; physical exam may reveal RUQ tenderness to palpation of the rib cage or abdomen itself; leukocytosis, increases in liver transaminases, anemia, and mild increase in alkaline phosphatase; plain films show right-sided atelectasis, elevated hemidiaphragm, pleural effusion, and perhaps a subdiaphragmatic air-fluid level

Diagnosis

▶ **Benign noncystic lesions** - may be confidently differentiated from each other and malignancies using ultrasound, helical CT, Tc-99m pertechnetate - labeled RBC, and MRI; biopsy and/or resection rarely necessary

▶ **Liver cysts**
   1. *Polycystic disease* - ultrasound and CT are useful for diagnosis and screening of other organs
   2. *Cystadenoma* - CT and, if necessary, enucleation for histologic examination
   3. *Hydatid liver cyst* - ultrasound and CT; skin testing (Casoni test) and serologic studies may be used as an adjunct.

▶ **Hepatocellular carcinoma** - serum alfa fetoprotein; ultrasound, CT, and MRI aid in diagnosis, staging, and surgical planning; biopsy is rarely necessary.

▶ **Hepatic abscess** - ultrasound and CT

Treatment

▶ **Benign noncystic liver lesions** - hemangiomas and focal nodular hyperplasia lesions do not need to be excised or resected; hepatic adenomas should undergo resection for intraperitoneal rupture or hemorrhage; oral contraceptives should be discontinued in patients suspected of having a hepatic adenoma; if there is no regression of the adenoma with oral contraceptive cessation, the adenoma should be excised.

▶ **Liver cysts**
   1. *polycystic disease* - asymptomatic lesions do not require excision; large, symptomatic lesions can be percutaneously aspirated and sclerosed with 95% ethanol; if there is a recurrence of cysts, surgical unroofing and decompression should be considered.
   2. *cystadenoma* - complete excision by either enucleation or liver resection

TABLE 14-1
IMAGING TECHNIQUES AND HEPATIC MASSES

Technique	Discussion
U/S	Noninvasive, low cost, readily available; with Doppler imaging, also provides information on vascular patency and volume and direction of flow; sensitivity to 1 cm; ideal screening technique; diagnostic for simple cysts; unable to convincingly determine etiology of solid or mixed masses; excellent technique for guided biopsy; marked obesity or bowel gas interferes with the examination; generally the screening test of first choice
CT	Radiation and contrast exposure; readily available and provides "normal anatomy" for nonradiologist; sensitivity to 1 cm; nearly isodense lesions may be missed due to volume averaging or timing of imaging to contrast injection; will screen for extrahepatic lesions simultaneously, thus identifying metastatic disease beyond the liver
Triphasic helical CT	Increased radiation exposure (must first localize lesion and then take multiple timed images); correctly identifies two-thirds of hemangiomas
CTAP	Invasive, requiring placement of angiography catheter for bolus injection; superior delineation of anatomic location of lesions to help with surgical planning; more sensitive than standard CT and will often save unnecessary surgery by identifying additional tumor nodules not noted on standard CT or US; may produce increase in false-positive findings in presence of severe cirrhosis
MRI	Totally noninvasive but very expensive; excellent biplanar images with sensitivity to 1.0 cm; more accurate than CTAP in the presence of severe cirrhosis; problems identifying lesions near the diaphragm due to cardiac motion-induced artifacts; provides additional information on vascular supply and patency
Angiography	Most invasive with high contrast dose and high radiation exposure; most expensive (along with MRI); provides most accurate information on vascular supply, patency, and flow, including pressures if needed
Nuclear medicine	Minimally invasive, less costly (except for US), and readily available; less sensitive (2.0 cm minimum); primarily useful to distinguish hepatic adenomas from focal nodular hyperplasia (due to the lack of Kupffer cells for colloid uptake in the adenomas) and identifying hemangiomas (with the Tc-99m-tagged RBC-SPECT study)[a]

[a]RBC-SPECT, Tc-99m-tagged red blood cell study utilizing single photon emission computed tomography.

3. *hydatid liver cysts* - complete surgical removal is required for cure; systemic medications, such as mebendazole or albendazole, may be used as an adjunct to surgery.

► **Hepatocellular carcinoma** - hepatic resection or liver transplant
► **Hepatic abscess -** antibiotics (metronidazole and ceftazidime or aztreonam) along with CT or ultrasound-guided percutaneous aspiration should be attempted first; failure of conservative management necessitates an open surgical intervention.

REFERENCES

1. Schwartz SI, Shires GT, Spencer FC, et al. *Principles of Surgery*. New York: McGraw-Hill, 1999.
2. Bland KI. *The Practice of General Surgery*. Philadelphia: WB Saunders, 2002.
3. Townsend CM, Beauchamp RD, Evers BM, et al. *Sabiston Textbook of Surgery: The Biologic Basis of Modern Surgical Practice*. Philadelphia: WB Saunders, 2001.

CHAPTER 15

MISCELLANEOUS HEPATOLOGY PEARLS

BENIGN RECURRENT INTRAHEPATIC CHOLESTASIS

► sx/signs - > 2 episodes of jaundice separated by sx-free period of months to years, recurs ~ q 2 years, history of jaundice in childhood, usually presents before age 30, jaundice preceded by severe pruritus, avg episode lasts 3 months, hallmark - marked ↑ in alk Φ which may be ≥1000, also see bili up to 10–15, GGT usually < 100, AST and ALT usually normally or just minimally elevated
► defect in bile acid transport and secretion with resultant contraction of bile acid pool secondary to increase in fecal bile acid loss
► autosomal recessive with gene defect on long arm of chromosome 18
► 50% with family h/o cholestasis
► most commonly seen in northern Mediterranean ancestry

WORK-UP OF ASCITES

► treatment of cirrhotic ascites:
  • diuretics: spironolactone (100 mg with max of 400 mg/day) + furosemide (40 mg with max of 160 mg/day)
  • large volume paracentesis: 4–6 L per session; if > 5 L removed, supplement with IV albumin 6–8 g/L removed
  • refractory ascites
    1. TIPS (transjugular intrahepatic portosystemic shunt)
    2. OLT (orthotopic liver transplant) - 70% response rate in ascites
► infected ascites:
  • The most common organism is gram-negative bacilli from intestinal origin, especially *E. coli.*

TABLE 15-1
WORK-UP OF ASCITES

SAAG[a] High gradient (> 1.1 g/dL)	SAAG[a] Low gradient (< 1.1 g/dL)
Cirrhosis Alcoholic hepatitis Cardiac ascites Massive liver mets Fulminant hepatic failure Budd-Chiari syndrome Portal vein thrombosis Veno-occlusive disease Acute fatty liver of pregnancy Myxedema "Mixed" ascites	Peritoneal carcinomatosis TB (without cirrhosis) Pancreatic ascites (without cirrhosis) Biliary ascites (without ascites) Nephrotic syndrome Connective tissue disease Bowel obstruction or infarction SAAG < 1.1 → no portal hypertension

[a]SAAG, serum-ascites albumin gradient = serum albumin – ascites albumin.

- treat until symptoms resolved and F/U PMN < 250 mm^3
- 40% 1-year survival in cirrhotic without transplantation
  - treatment regimens:
    1. antibiotic of choice - IV cefotaxime (or other 3rd generation cephalosporin)
    2. other options - ofloxacin 400 mg po bid, IV amoxicillin-clavulanic acid
    3. prophylaxis after first episode - 400 mg po per day norfloxacin

TABLE 15-2
WORK-UP OF ASCITES

Category of infection	Ascitic fluid analysis
SBP	PMN ≥ 250/mm^3, single organism; 500 WBc/cc ascites
Culture-negative neutrocytic ascites	PMN ≥ 250/mm^3, negative culture
Secondary bacterial peritonitis	PMN ≥ 250/mm^3, usually multiple organisms; glucose, 50 mg/dL, LDH[a] > serum level LDH, TP[b] > 1g/dL
Monomicrobial bacterascites	PMN < 250/mm^3, single organism
Polymicrobial bacterascites	PMN < 250/mm^3, multiple organisms

[a]LDH, lactate dehydrogenase; [b]TP, total protein.

► evaluation of ascitic fluid:
  • portal hypertension: clear yellow fluid
  • infection: cloudy fluid; need ≥10,000 organisms/mL for positive gram stain
  • chylous: milky fluid; triglycerides > 200 mg/dL
  • malignant: red tint (implies ≥10,000 RBC/µL), bloody fluid
  • pancreatic: tea-colored or black fluid
  • SBP: polys ≥ 250 cells/µL and represents > 50% of total WBC
  • biliary or bowel perforation: ascites triglycerides > serum triglycerides

PORTAL GASTROPATHY/COLOPATHY
► common, variable course
► bleeding uncommon
► severity correlates with severity of liver disease
► ↑ risk with previous sclerotherapy or EVL
► effective for both esophageal and gastric varices

VARICES
► seen in 5–15% of cirrhotics
► avg lifetime risk of bleeding 30%
► 20–30% mortality rate with each bleeding episode
► 50% mortality rate with first bleeding episode
► primary prophylaxis - nonselective β-blocker (propranolol, nadolol); ? combination with NTG more efficacious
► secondary prophylaxis - EVL more effective than sclerotherapy and has fewer side effects, TIPS

HEPATORENAL SYNDROME (HRS)
► treatment of choice - OLT
► for dx, must exclude: (1) recent exposure to nephrotoxic agents, (2) shock preceding onset of HRS, (3) active bacterial infection, (4) significant proteinuria (> 500 mg/dL) and/or ultrasonographic evidence of renal abnormalities

HEPATOPULMONARY SYNDROME

▶ triad - liver disease + hypoxemia (O_2 < 70 or alveolar-arterial O_2 gradient of > 20 mm Hg) + intrapulmonary vascular dilations (as dx'd on contrast-enhanced echo)
▶ can be seen in any Child's class
▶ can be seen in presence or absence of portal hypertension
▶ mortality rate up to 40%
▶ cause of death - GIB, sepsis, renal failure

ACUTE/FULMINANT HEPATIC FAILURE

▶ Rx-induced etiology responsible for 33% of cases
▶ ↑ risk from Rx:
  • INH, valproate, halothane, phenytoin
  • rifampin + INH
  • rifampin + pyrazinamide
  • ETOH + acetaminophen (may see ↑↑↑ of AST and ALT up to 30K)
  • acetaminophen + INH
  • TMP-SMX
▶ path - massive hepatocyte necrosis, microvesicular fat
▶ may be initial presentation of (previously unrecognized):
  • Wilson's disease (often with intravascular hemolysis)
  • autoimmune chronic hepatitis
  • HBV reactivation or HBeAg seroconversion flare
  • HDV superinfection in HBV carrier
  • HAV superinfection in asxtic CLD
▶ cause of death - cerebral edema > renal failure > bleeding
▶ 1-year OLT survival = 75%; 5-year = 60–65%

ORTHOTOPIC LIVER TRANSPLANT (OLT)

▶ **Complications:**
  • hypertension in 70% related to immunosuppressive Rx and exacerbated by ACE inhibitors
  • renal insufficiency seen in 25–65% and related to immunosuppressive Rx and exacerbated by NSAIDs and ACE inhibitors, may be seen in immediate posttransplant period or insidiously between 1–2 years after, may progress to need for dialysis or renal transplant in 15%

- malignancy: ↑ risk of skin ca (squamous and basal cell; risk increases with duration of immunosuppressive Rx), lymphoma, Kaposi sarcoma
- infection: CMV hepatitis/chorioretinitis/myocarditis/colitis/pneumonitis, fungal, pneumocystic pneumonia
- Rx toxicities:
  a. cyclosporine - hirsutism, ↑ cholesterol, neuropathy, gingival hyperplasia, HTN, gout, CRI
  b. tacrolimus (FK506) - hair loss, diabetes, HTN, CRI
- Rx interactions with cyclosporine and tacrolimus:
  a. NSAIDs → renal insufficiency
  b. ACE inhibitors → renal insufficiency
  c. HMG CoA inhibitors → rhabdomyolysis
  d. allopurinol + azathioprine → aplastic anemia
  e. erythromycin, diltiazem, → ↑ cyclosporine and FK506 levels
  f. ketoconazole → ↑ cyclosporine level
- allograft rejection:
  1. *acute* - seen in 30–70% within first 6 months, ↑ AST/ALT/bili; liver bx: bile duct destruction, lymphs
  2. *chronic* - seen in 5–10%, common indication for re-transplantation, chronic ↑ alk Φ and bili; liver bx: vanishing bile duct syndrome
  3. *biliary tract* - stricture, leak
- headache
- obesity
▶ usual cause of death:
  - fulminant hepatitis - life support issues
  - hemochromatosis - infection and cardiac problems
  - HCC - recurrent disease

CANCER

▶ cholangiocarcinoma - $2/3$ perihilar, $1/4$ distal extrahepatic, remainder intrahepatic, including Klatskin (bifurcation of hepatic duct)
▶ liver ca - 98% metastatic disease; 2% primary liver ca - HCC, cholangiocarcinoma
▶ HCC paraneoplastic syndromes:
  - hypoglycemia
  - erythrocytosis (polycythemia)

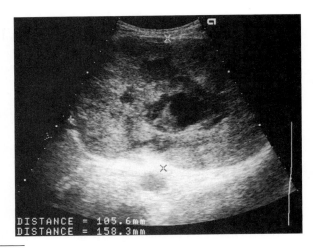

FIGURE 15-1
Ultrasound of HCC. (Reproduced with permission from Friedman SL, McQuaid KR, Grendell JH. *Current Diagnosis & Treatment in Gastroenterology*. Lange Medical Books/ McGraw-Hill, 2003.)

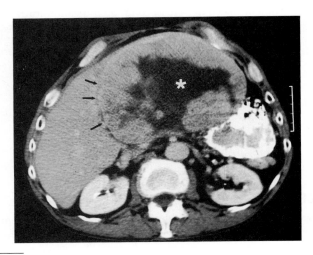

FIGURE 15-2
CT scan of HCC. (Reproduced with permission from Friedman SL, McQuaid KR, Grendell JH. *Current Diagnosis & Treatment in Gastroenterology*. Lange Medical Books/ McGraw-Hill, 2003.)

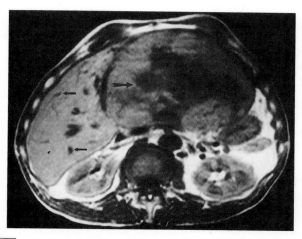

FIGURE 15-3
MRI of HCC. (Reproduced with permission from Friedman SL, McQuaid KR, Grendell JH. *Current Diagnosis & Treatment in Gastroenterology*. Lange Medical Books/McGraw-Hill, 2003.)

- hypercalcemia
- watery diarrhea syndrome: secretory, hypokalemia, achlorhydria; prostaglandin E2/VIP/gastrin detected in tumor
- symptomatic porphyria (porphyria cutanea tarda symptomatica): light-sensitive dermatosis; porphyrin excretion not consistent with any of the inherited porphyrias
- sexual changes: isosexual precocity, gynecomastia, feminization
- systemic arterial hypertension
- carcinoid syndrome
- hypertrophic osteoarthropathy
- osteoporosis/osteopenia
- skin rashes

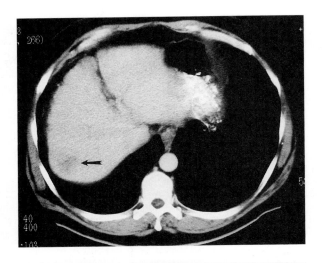

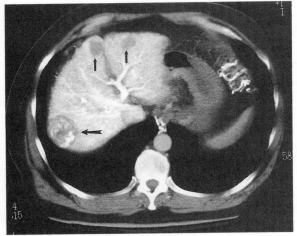

FIGURE 15-4

CTAP of HCC. (Reproduced with permission from Friedman SL, McQuaid KR, Grendell JH. *Current Diagnosis & Treatment in Gastroenterology.* Lange Medical Books/ McGraw-Hill, 2003.)

TABLE 15-3
CANCER DEMOGRAPHICS

Feature	Fibrolamellar ca	HCC
Avg age	23	55–60
Gender	Male = female	Male:female = 4:1
Cirrhosis	4%	80%
Cure rate	32%	0–34%
Survival	43 mos	6.5 mos

TABLE 15-4
FREQUENCY OF TUMOR METASTASIS TO LIVER[a]

Primary tumor	Percent with liver metastasis
Gallbladder	77.6
Pancreas	70.4
Unknown primary	57.0
Colon	56.0
Breast	53.2
Melanoma	50.0
Ovary	48.0
Stomach	44.0
Bronchogenic	41.8

[a]Data derived from Craig JR, Peters RL, Edmondson HA. *Tumors of the Liver and the Intrahepatic Bile Ducts.* Armed Forces Institutes of Pathology, 1989:257.

REFERENCES

1. Ostapowicz G, Fontana RJ, Schiodt FV, et al. Results of a prospective study of acute liver failure at 17 tertiary care centers in the United States. *Ann Intern Med* 2002;137:947–954.
2. Arroyo V, Guevara M, Gines P. Hepatorenal syndrome in cirrhosis: pathogenesis and treatment. *Gastroenterology* 2002;122:1658–1676.
3. Boyer TD. Transjugular intrahepatic portosystemic shunt: current status. *Gastroenterology* 2003;124:1700–1710.
4. Narayanan Menon KV, Gores GJ, Shah VH. Pathogenesis, diagnosis, and treatment of alcoholic liver disease. *Mayo Clin Proc* 2001;76:1021–1029.
5. Maddrey WC. Update in hepatology. *Ann Intern Med* 2001;134(3):216–223.
6. Lewis JH, guest ed. Drug-induced liver disease. In: *Gastroenterology Clinics of North America.* Philadelphia: WB Saunders, December 1995.
7. Bacon BR, DiBisceglie AM. *Liver Disease Diagnosis and Management.* Philadelphia: Churchill Livingstone, 2000.

8. Edwards ZC. Gastroenterology. In: Edwards TI, Mayer T, eds. *Urgent Care Medicine*. New York: McGraw-Hill, 2002:327.

9. McNally PR. *GI/Liver Secrets*. 2nd ed. Philadelphia: Hanley & Belfus, 2001.

10. Tran TT, Poordad FF, Nissen N, Martin P. Hepatocellular carcinoma: an update. *Clin Perspect Gastroenterol* 2002;5(5):302–306.

11. Schilsky ML. Wilson's disease. *Clin Perspect Gastroenterol* 2002;(4):234–243.

12. DiBisceglie AM. Hepatocellular carcinoma. *Clin Perspect Gastroenterol* 2000;3(1):33–39.

13. Ko CW, Lee SP. Gallbladder disease. *Clin Perspect Gastroenterol* 2000;3(2):87–96.

14. Wiesner RH, Rakela J, Ishitani MB, et al. Recent advances in liver transplantation. *Mayo Clin Proc* 2003;78:197–210.

15. Brown RS, guest ed. Endoscopic issues in liver transplantation. In: *Gastrointestinal Endoscopy Clinics of North America*. Philadelphia: WB Saunders, January 2001.

16. Cheng SJ, Pratt DS. Liver transplantation. *Clin Perspect Gastroenterol* 2002;5(4):221–228.

17. Collins J, Corless CL, Deveney K. Pouchitis. *Clin Perspect Gastroenterol* 2002;5(3):156–161.

18. Van Thiel H, DeMaria N, Brems JJ, et al. Liver transplantation: what the non-hepatologist should know. *Pract Gastroenterol* 2001;XXV(4):42–66.

CHAPTER 16

THE BILIARY TREE

BILIARY TREE
Highlights

▶ **Origin of Symptoms:**
- Symptoms are a result of biliary tract obstruction, infection, or both.
- Obstruction can be extramural (pancreatic cancer), intramural (cholangiocarcinoma), or intraluminal (choledocholithiasis).
- Infection within the biliary tree requires a susceptible host, a sufficient inoculum, and stasis.
- Scleral icterus develops when the serum bilirubin reaches a concentration of approximately 2.5 mg/dL.
- Jaundice develops when the serum bilirubin levels exceeds 5 mg/dL.

▶ **Major Syndromes:**
- calculous disease
- acalculous cholecystitis
- recurrent pyogenic cholangitis
- Mirizzi's syndrome
- neoplasms

Demographics

▶ **Calculous disease** - 40 years of age with a female:male ratio = 3:1; increased relative risk if parents, siblings, or 1st degree relatives have calculous disease; other risk factors are obesity, TPN, and Crohn's disease; associated with intestinal bypass surgery and low-calorie, high-protein diets

▶ **Acalculous cholecystitis** - fasting critically ill or septic patients (usually found in the intensive care unit); acute transmural inflammation of the gallbladder in the absence of gallstones; pathogenesis is the result of gallbladder ischemia.

▶ **Recurrent pyogenic cholangitis** - also known as oriental cholangiohepatitis; endemic to Southeast Asia; number one cause of acute abd pain in Hong Kong emergency rooms; the characteristic ductal ectasia and stricture along with intrahepatic stone formation may be caused by parasitic infections (*Clonorchis sinensis* and/or *Ascaris lumbricoides*), indolent bacterial infections, and protein malnutrition.

▶ **Mirizzi's syndrome** - more prevalent in the elderly, but can occur in any patient with cholelithiasis; obstruction of the common bile duct by a stone in the cystic duct or Hartmann's pouch; a long cystic duct running parallel to the common duct or a low cystic-common duct junction predispose to this condition; type I: hepatic duct is compressed by a large stone impacted in the cystic duct or Hartmann's pouch; type II: the stone has eroded into the hepatic duct, producing a cholecystocholedochal fistula.

▶ **Neoplasms:**
  • *gallbladder cancer:* most common biliary system malignancy; 5th most common GI tract cancer; 1% of all cancers; 2 to 3 cases per 100,000 persons in the U.S.; women outnumber men 3 to 1; mean age is the 7th decade of life; high-risk groups include Native Americans, Israelis, Chileans, Poles, Japanese, Bolivians, and Mexicans; associated with cholelithiasis, chronic cholecystitis, exposure to industrial carcinogens, gallbladder adenomas, and IBD
  • *cholangiocarcinoma:* overall incidence of 1 per 100,000 persons; equal frequency among women and men; incidence increases with age; high-risk groups include Native Americans, Israelis, and Japanese; etiology related to chronic inflammation, gallstones, and stasis within the biliary system; risk factors are UC, PSC, and choledochal cysts
  • *choledochal cysts:* benign neoplasm; predominantly affects women; postulated etiology is an anomalous junction of the common bile and pancreatic ducts with resultant chronic reflux of biliopancreatic secretions
  • *biliary polyps:* benign neoplasm; arise most often from the columnar epithelium lining of the gallbladder; may arise

from the supporting muscle and fibrous tissue of the gall-bladder; may be sessile or pedunculated; may be capable of malignant degeneration

Symptoms/Signs/Labs

▶ **Calculous disease:**
   • *acute cholecystitis:* initial pain is vague and visceral, but intensifies and localizes to the RUQ over time; patient may complain of N&V, anorexia, and low-grade fever; guarding, rebound tenderness, a palpable mass in the RUQ, and positive Murphy's sign (inspiratory arrest on palpation of the RUQ) may be appreciated on physical exam; mild leukocytosis and minor elevations in liver function tests
   • *choledocholithiasis:* may produce a variety of symptoms including jaundice, cholangitis, acute pancreatitis, or systemic sepsis; elevated bilirubin and alk phos
   • *cholangitis:* Charcot's triad (RUQ abd pain, jaundice, fever); may progress to the Pentad of Reynolds (Charcot's triad plus altered mental status and hypotension)
   • *gallstone ileus:* results from a gallstone ≥ 2 cm in diameter passing through a cholecystoduodenal fistula and becoming lodged in the terminal ileum (the narrowest segment of bowel), creating a small bowel obstruction; typical patient is an elderly woman with a history of biliary colic presenting with a "tumbling" bowel obstruction

▶ **Acalculous cholecystitis** - usually complicated by gangrene, empyema, and perforation

▶ **Recurrent pyogenic cholangitis** - abd pain, fever, and presence of intrahepatic and extrahepatic pigment stones in the absence of disease within the gallbladder; jaundice is uncommon due to segmental (not complete) bile duct obstruction; recurring episodes over years to decades with the patient seeking medical attention only when the frequency and severity of the attacks become intolerable

▶ **Mirizzi's syndrome** - painless jaundice or cholangitis, depending on the presence of contaminated bile

▶ **Neoplasms** - clinically silent tumors that only become symptomatic when they have reached an advanced stage of development and are usually incurable; painless jaundice, weight loss, nausea, anorexia, fatigue, back pain, and a host of other nonspecific symptoms

Diagnosis

▶ **Calculous disease:**
   - *acute cholecystitis:* abd U/S demonstrating gallbladder wall thickening and pericholecystic fluid; ultrasonographer may demonstrate a "sonographic Murphy's sign"
   - *choledocholithiasis:* high suspicion in a patient with cholangitis, common bile duct stones on U/S, or preoperative jaundice; definitively identified by cholangiography
   - *cholangitis:* percutaneous transhepatic cholangiography when U/S shows a dilated proximal duct system or ERCP when the duct system is normal on U/S (these procedures should be done following the acute phase of the disease)
   - *gallstone ileus:* suspect in patients presenting with bowel obstruction in the absence of an incarcerated hernia or a history of prior abd surgery; may see a large mass at the site of the bowel obstruction and air in the biliary tree; U/S may be helpful

▶ **Acalculous cholecystitis** - high suspicion, as most patients are sedated and unable to provide a history or participate in the physical exam; cholescintigraphy, U/S, and percutaneous aspiration of bile showing the presence of bacteria and leukocytes

▶ **Recurrent pyogenic cholangitis** - history and physical exam

▶ **Mirizzi's syndrome** - dx usually made during cholecystectomy

▶ **Neoplasms** - CT and angiography; ERCP may be used to obtain brushings to diagnose cholangiocarcinoma

Treatment

▶ **Calculous disease:**
   - *acute cholecystitis:* cholecystectomy and antibiotic therapy directed toward enteric bacteria (ampicillin/gentamicin combination or a 2nd generation cephalosporin) begun on admission and continued 24 hours postoperatively
   - *choledocholithiasis:* ERCP with sphincterotomy and stone extraction should be attempted first; laparoscopic and/or open choledocholithotomy
   - *cholangitis:* ampicillin, an aminoglycoside, and either clindamycin or metronidazole should be started immediately; once the patient has been afebrile for 48 hours, treatment of the underlying disorder can begin

- *gallstone ileus:* exploratory laparotomy to remove the stone; removal of the gallbladder is not advised
► **Acalculous cholecystitis** - emergency cholecystectomy or percutaneous cholecystostomy in high-risk patients
► **Recurrent pyogenic cholangitis** - decompression of the obstructed bile ducts and removal of as many stones and intraluminal debris as possible
► **Mirizzi's syndrome** - type I: cholecystectomy; type II: partial cholecystectomy and bilioenteric anastomosis
► **Neoplasms -** curative resection may be attempted in gallbladder cancers and cholangiocarcinomas classified as stage I or stage II; stage III and stage IV carcinomas are treated with palliation; choledochal cysts are best treated with complete excision and Roux-en-Y hepaticojejunostomy

REFERENCES

1. Norton JA, Bollinger RR, Chang AE, et al. *Surgery, Basic Science and Clinical Evidence.* New York: Springer-Verlag, 2001.
2. Schwartz SI, Shires GT, Spencer FC, et al. *Principles of Surgery.* New York: McGraw-Hill, 1999.
3. Bland KI. *The Practice of General Surgery.* Philadelphia: WB Saunders, 2002.
4. Townsend CM, Beauchamp RD, Evers BM, et al. *Sabiston Textbook of Surgery: The Biologic Basis of Modern Surgical Practice.* Philadelphia: WB Saunders, 2001.

PART III

THE PANCREAS

CHAPTER 17

THE PANCREAS

PANCREAS

Highlights

▶ The pancreas is composed of exocrine tissue (acinar cells), endocrine tissue (islets of Langerhans), and connective tissue.

▶ The exocrine portion of the gland produces amylase, lipase, trypsin, chymotrypsin, deoxyribonuclease, and ribonuclease. Duct cells produce bicarbonate.

▶ Intracellular calcium is the most important determinant of enzyme secretion.

▶ Somatostatin inhibits pancreatic exocrine secretion.

▶ Secretin controls bicarbonate and fluid secretion.

▶ Cholecystokinin (CCK) stimulates pancreatic exocrine secretion.

▶ The islets of Langerhans are composed of alpha, beta, and delta cells.

▶ The endocrine portion of the gland produces insulin, glucagon, somatostatin, and pancreatic polypeptide.

▶ Glucagon is produced in the alpha cells, insulin in the beta cells, and somatostatin in the delta cells.

▶ An elevated amylase without pancreatitis suggests a differential diagnosis which includes organ rupture, CRI/CRF, and mumps.

▶ **Major Syndromes:**
  • acute pancreatitis
  • chronic pancreatitis
  • pancreatic pseudocysts
  • pancreatic cancer
  • cystic tumors

TABLE 17-1
PANCREATIC ENZYMES FOR THE TREATMENT OF STEATORRHEA[a] OR PAIN[b]

Brand name	Units of lipase per pill
Conventional enzyme preparations	
Viokase, Viokase 16	8000, 16,000
Ku-Zyme HP	8000
Generic pancrelipase	8000
Enteric-coated enzyme preparations	
Creon 5, 10, 20	5000, 10,000, 20,000
Pancrease MT 4, 10, 16, 20	4000, 10,000, 16,000, 20,000
Ultrase, Ultrase MT 12, 18, 20	4500, 12,000, 18,000, 20,000

[a]For the treatment of steatorrhea, both conventional and enteric-coated preparations can be used. The dosage depends on the lipase content. 30,000 units of lipase should be delivered with each meal. Low-potency formulations (5000–8000 units of lipase per pill) require four to six pills with each meal. Higher potency formulations require two to three pills with each meal. Conventional enzymes require co-treatment with agents to suppress gastric acid.
[b]For the treatment of pain, conventional enzyme preparations are used, four to eight pills (depending on potency) before meals and at night. An adjuvant agent to reduce gastric acid is required, either H2-receptor antagonists or a proton-pump inhibitor.

Demographics

► **Acute pancreatitis** - etiologic factors include cholelithiasis (45%), ETOH (35%), idiopathic (10%), and miscellaneous [10%; includes hypertensive sphincter of Oddi dysfunction, pancreas divisum, microlithiasis, hyperlipidemia (need triglycerides in the 700–1000 range, with 500 as the threshold for consideration), hypercalcemia, trauma, pancreatic ischemia, various drugs (azathioprine/6-MP, valproate, estrogen, thiazide, pentamidine/DDI, furosemide, sulfonamides), infection, toxins, and perhaps genetics]; may be mild or severe, with an overall mortality rate of 10% and complication rate of 25%; early (first 7 days) complications: uni- or multi-organ failure from shock and pulmonary insufficiency, DIC, hypocalcemia, hyperglycemia; late (after 7 days) complications: pseudocyst, abscess or infected necrosis (40–50% infection rate), pseudoaneurysm and bleeding, DIC, splenic infarction

► **Chronic pancreatitis** - most cases are the result of excessive alcohol intake; also seen in conjunction with hyperparathyroidism, cystic fibrosis, and pancreatic duct anomalies; gallstone disease does not result in chronic pancreatitis; irreversible parenchymal destruction occurs within the pancreatic tissue;

endocrine insufficiency results after 80% of the gland is destroyed; exocrine insufficiency results after 90% of the gland is destroyed; hereditary pancreatitis: autosomal dominant, gene mutation on chromosome 7q - cationic trypsinogen; abnormal secretin test indicates 60% damage, ERCP changes and calcifications on CT suggest 60–85% damage, and diabetes/malabsorption indicates > 90% damage.

▶ **Pancreatic pseudocysts** - occur in up to 10% of patients with acute or chronic pancreatitis; contain high levels of the pancreatic enzymes amylase, lipase, and trypsin; lack an epithelial lining; may be complicated by infection

▶ **Pancreatic cancer** - 3% of all cancers and 5% of all cancer deaths; 5-year survival rate is 3%; 90% of patients die within the 1st year of diagnosis; risk factors include smoking, chronic pancreatitis, diabetes mellitus, prior gastrectomy, and a high fat diet; mutation of the K-*ras* oncogene present in a majority of cases; 90% of the exocrine tumors are adenocarcinomas; two-thirds of the adenocarcinomas are found within the head of the pancreas.

▶ **Cystic tumors** - represent 20% of cystic lesions found in the pancreas (the other 80% are pseudocysts); cyst wall contains an epithelial lining; most are benign; mucinous cystic neoplasms and cystadenocarcinoma, and intraductal papillary mucinous tumors have malignant potential.

Symptoms/Signs/Labs

▶ **Acute pancreatitis** - diffuse abd pain radiating to the back; pain is severe and steady; nausea, vomiting, hypotension, tachycardia, fever, epigastric tenderness, abd distention; severe cases may involve hemorrhage and produce Grey Turner's sign (ecchymoses of the flanks) or Cullen's sign (ecchymoses of the periumbilical region); elevated serum amylase, lipase, WBC count, LFTs, and hyperglycemia; may see a decrease in serum calcium and serum albumin; the higher the AST and ALT the greater the likelihood of gallstones as the etiology; if amylase is elevated but ≤ 3× normal and lipase is elevated, check trypsinogen to verify acute pancreatitis.

▶ **Chronic pancreatitis** - epigastric abd pain radiating to the back, nausea, anorexia, weight loss; serum amylase, lipase, and LFTs may be mildly elevated or normal; trypsinogen < 10 ng/mL indicates exocrine insufficiency

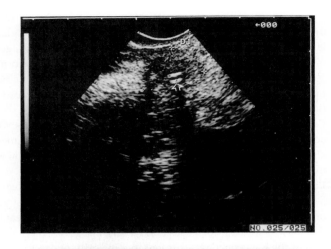

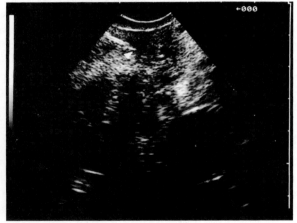

FIGURE 17-1
Endoscopic ultrasound (EUS) of pancreatic cancer. (Reproduced with permission from Friedman SL, McQuaid KR, Grendell JH. *Current Diagnosis & Treatment in Gastroenterology.* Lange Medical Books/McGraw-Hill, 2003.)

▶ **Pancreatic pseudocyst** - upper abd pain, N&V, early satiety, and weight loss; abd tenderness, a palpable abd mass, fever, jaundice, and ascites may be appreciated on exam; look for signs of hemorrhage and infection; may have slightly elevated serum amylase and LFTs

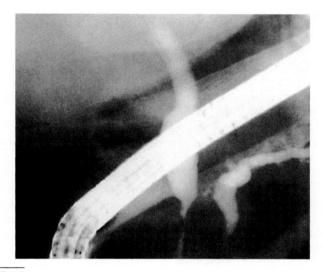

FIGURE 17-2
ERCP of "double duct" sign of pancreatic head carcinoma. (Reproduced with permission from Friedman SL, McQuaid KR, Grendell JH. *Current Diagnosis & Treatment in Gastroenterology*. Lange Medical Books/McGraw-Hill, 2003.)

▶ **Pancreatic cancer** - most patients have advanced disease at time of presentation; painless or a dull visceral pain radiating to the back, ascites, jaundice, cola-colored urine, clay-colored stools, and pruritus; marked elevation of serum bilirubin and mild elevation of hepatic transaminases; Courvoisier's sign (palpable gallbladder in the right midclavicular line at the costal margin); Virchow's node (lymphadenopathy in the left supraclavicular fossa); Sister Mary Joseph's node (lymphadenopathy in the periumbilical region); Blumer's shelf (pelvic tumor palpable on rectal exam)

▶ **Cystic tumors** - may have vague abd pain, bloating, weight loss; many are incidental findings; dilated pancreatic duct and steatorrhea in 33–47% of cases of mucinous cystadenoma; septated, calcified pancreatic cyst is suggestive of cystadenoma (malignant); indolent course, a high rate of malignant transformation and a dilated pancreatic duct are seen with an intraductal papillary mucinous tumor (mucinous ductal ectasia).

Diagnosis

▶ **Acute pancreatitis** - hyperamylasemia, elevated lipase; U/S to evaluate for gallstones; sentinel loop sign (dilated proximal jejunal loop in the upper abd close to the pancreatic bed); colon cutoff sign (distention of the colon to the level of the transverse colon, with sparse air in the splenic flexure and distal colon); severity of disease can be assessed using the Ranson criteria or the APACHE-II severity of disease classification system; CT if pancreatic necrosis is suspected; ERCP to evaluate structural causes and remove stones in gallstone pancreatitis

▶ **Chronic pancreatitis** - plain films may show pancreatic calcifications (calcifications are a hallmark of chronic pancreatitis, but the extent of calcification does not correlate with the extent of exocrine insufficiency); "chain of lakes" (ductal dilatation and ductal stricturing) seen on endoscopic retrograde cholangiopancreatography; CT may show the extent of glandular destruction; secretin test in which all 4 bicarbonate collections are > 80 is abnormal and suggests chronic pancreatitis; trypsinogen ≤ 20 ng/mL indicates exocrine insufficiency and ≤ 10 ng/mL indicates severe exocrine insufficiency.

```
Ranson/Imrie criteria
    At admission or diagnosis
        Age >55 years
        Leukocytosis >16,000/μL
        Hyperglycemia >11 mmol/L (> 200 mg/dL)
        Serum LDH >400 IU/L
        Serum AST >250 IU/L
    During initial 48 h
        Fall in hematocrit by >10 percent
        Fluid deficit of >4000 mL
        Hypocalcemia [calcium concentration <1.9 mmol/L (<8.0 mg/dL)]
        Hypoxemia (P$_{O2}$ <60 mmHg)
        Increase in BUN to >1.8 mmol/L (>5 mg/dL) after IV fluid administration
        Hypoalbuminemia [albumin level <32 g/L (<3.2 g/dL)]
Acute physiology and chronic health evaluation (APACHE II) score >12
Hemorrhagic peritoneal fluid
Obesity [body mass index (BMI) >29]
Key indicators of organ failure
    Hypotension (blood pressure <90 mmHg) or tachycardia >130 beats per minute
    P$_{O2}$ <60 mmHg
    Oliguria (<50 mL/h) or increasing blood urea nitrogen (BUN), creatinine
    Metabolic indicators: serum calcium <1.9 mmol/L (<8.0 mg/dL) or
        serum albumin <32 g/L (<3.2 g/dL)
```

FIGURE 17-3

Ranson-Imrie criteria. (Reproduced with permission from Braunwald E, Fauci AS, Kasper DL, et al. *Harrison's Principles of Internal Medicine.* 16th ed. McGraw-Hill, 2005.)

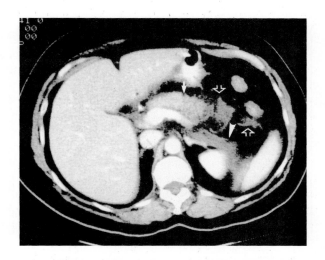

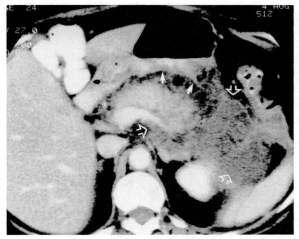

FIGURE 17-4

CT scan of acute pancreatitis. (Reproduced with permission from Braunwald E, Fauci AS, Kasper DL, et al. *Harrison's Principles of Internal Medicine.* 15th ed. McGraw-Hill, 2001.)

TABLE 17-2
TESTS USEFUL IN THE DIAGNOSIS OF ACUTE AND CHRONIC PANCREATITIS AND PANCREATIC TUMORS

Test	Principle	Comment
Pancreatic enzymes in body fluids		
Amylase		
1. Serum	Pancreatic inflammation leads to increased enzyme levels	Simple: 20–40% false negatives and positives; reliable if test results are 3× the upper limit of normal
2. Urine	Renal clearance of amylase is increased in acute pancreatitis	May be abnormal when serum levels normal; false negatives and positives
3. Amylase/creatinine clearance ratio (C_{am}/C_{cr})	Renal clearance of amylase > clearance of creatinine	No more sensitive than serum amylase; many false positives
4. Ascitic fluid	Disruption of gland or main pancreatic duct leads to increased amylase concentration	Can establish diagnosis of pancreatitis; false positives occur with intestinal obstruction and perforated ulcer
5. Pleural fluid	Exudative pleural effusion with pancreatitis	False positives occur with carcinoma of the lung and esophageal perforation
6. Isoenzymes	P isoamylases arise from the pancreas; S isoamylases are from other sources	More sensitive than total serum amylase in diagnosis of acute pancreatitis; useful in identifying nonpancreatic causes of hyperamylasemia
Serum lipase	Pancreatic inflammation leads to increased enzyme levels	New methods have greatly simplified determination; positive in 70–85% of cases
Serum trypsinogen	Pancreatic inflammation leads to increased levels	*Elevated* in acute pancreatitis; *decreased* in chronic pancreatitis *with* steatorrhea; normal in chronic pancreatitis *without* steatorrhea and in steatorrhea with normal pancreatic function

Pancreatic polypeptide (PP)	PP confined almost totally to the pancreas; release stimulated by nutrients and hormones; such release parallels pancreatic enzyme secretion	Basal, meal-simulated, and hormone-stimulated [by secretin or cholecystokinin (CCK)] PP levels *decreased* in chronic pancreatitis, a fasting PP level > 125 pg/mL argues against chronic pancreatitis and pancreatic ca; increased levels in pancreatic endocrine tumors
Studies pertaining to pancreatic structure		
Radiologic and radionuclide tests 1. Plain film of the abdomen	Abnormal in acute and chronic pancreatitis	Simple; normal in > 50% of cases of both acute and chronic pancreatitis
2. Upper GI x-rays	Abnormally thickened duodenal folds; displacement of stomach or widening of duodenal loop suggests a pancreatic mass (inflammatory, neoplastic, cystic)	Simple; frequently normal; largely superseded by US and CT scanning
3. US	Can provide information on edema, inflammation, calcification, pseudocysts, and mass lesions	Simple, noninvasive; sequential studies quite feasible; useful in diagnosis of pseudocyst
4. CT scan	Permits detailed visualization of pancreas and surrounding structures	Useful in the diagnosis of pancreatic calcification, dilated pancreatic ducts, and pancreatic tumors; may not be able to distinguish between inflammatory and neoplastic mass lesions
5. Selective angiography	Can identify pancreatic neoplasms (1) by sheathing of celiac or superior mesenteric branches by tumor or (2) by tumor staining; displacement of vessels by tumor	Indicated (1) in suspected islet cell tumors and (2) before pancreatic or duodenal resection; most reliable features reflect nonresectable pancreatic ca

continued

TABLE 17-2
TESTS USEFUL IN THE DIAGNOSIS OF ACUTE AND CHRONIC PANCREATITIS AND PANCREATIC TUMORS (CONTINUED)

Test	Principle	Comment
6. Endoscopic retrograde cholangiopancreatography (ERCP)	Cannulation of pancreatic and common bile duct permits visualization of pancreatic-biliary ductal system	Provides diagnostic data in 60–85% of cases; differentiation of chronic pancreatitis from pancreatic carcinoma may be difficult
7. Endoscopic ultrasonography (EUS)	High-frequency transducer employed with EUS can produce very high-resolution images and depict changes in the pancreatic duct and parenchyma with better detail	Exact role of EUS vs. ERCP and CT not yet fully defined; sensitivity and specificity under study
8. MR cholangiopancreatography	Three-dimensional rendering has been used to produce very good images of the pancreatic duct by a noninvasive technique	May be used to evaluate patients judged to be at high risk for ERCP, such as the elderly; may replace ERCP as a diagnostic test, although large controlled studies need to be done
Pancreatic biopsy with US or CT guidance	Percutaneous biopsy with skinny needle and localization of lesion by US	High diagnostic yield; laparotomy avoided; requires special technical skills
Tests of exocrine pancreatic function		
Direct stimulation of the pancreas with analysis of duodenal contents		
1. Secretin-pancreozymin (CCK) test	Secretin leads to increased output of pancreatic juice and HCO_3^-; CCK leads to increased output of pancreatic enzymes; pancreatic secretory response is related to the functional mass of pancreatic tissue	Sensitive enough to detect occult disease; involves duodenal intubation and fluoroscopy; poorly defined normal enzyme response; overlap in chronic pancreatitis; large secretory reserve capacity of the pancreas

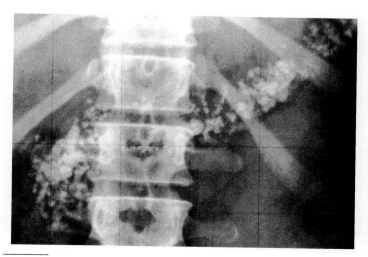

FIGURE 17-5
Pancreatic calcifications. (Reproduced with permission from Baker SR, Cho KC. *The Abdominal Plain Film with Correlative Imaging.* 2nd ed. Appleton & Lange, 1999.)

▶ **Pancreatic pseudocyst** - CT; U/S can be used during F/U to monitor interval size change.

▶ **Pancreatic cancer** - U/S is a useful screening tool to differentiate between gallstone disease and malignancy. An oral and IV contrast-enhanced, thin cut, spiral CT allows definitive identification and staging of the tumor. ERCP can be used to obtain brushings and define the biliary anatomy for future biliary-enteric reconstruction. Tumor marker CA 19-9 may be used during F/U to track disease state.

▶ **Cystic tumors**
  • *mucinous cystic neoplasms:* contain a tall columnar epithelium; stains positively for carcinoembryonic antigen (CEA); does not communicate with pancreatic duct
  • *cystadenocarcinoma:* contains a disordered columnar cell epithelium and papillary features
  • *intraductal papillary mucinous tumors:* ERCP is the key to diagnosis and shows mucin protruding through the papilla, dilated and irregular ducts, and filling defects within the ducts.

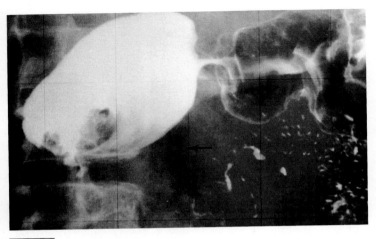

FIGURE 17-6
Pancreato-colic fistula. (Reproduced with permission from Baker SR, Cho KC. *The Abdominal Plain Film with Correlative Imaging.* 2nd ed. Appleton & Lange, 1999.)

Treatment

▶ **Acute pancreatitis** - patients with mild to moderate disease can be treated with IVF resuscitation, electrolyte replacement, pain medication (meperidine is preferred, as morphine may cause spasm in the sphincter of Oddi and exacerbate symptoms), and nasogastric suctioning for intractable vomiting. Prophylactic antibiotics should be added along with the appropriate supportive care for patients with severe pancreatitis (3 or more Ranson criteria with CT evidence of necrosis). Infected pancreatic necrosis (diagnosed by CT-guided fine-needle aspiration with Gram stain and culture) should be treated with IV antibiotics and immediate surgical debridement; otherwise surgery is indicated to establish diagnosis or correct biliary disease (i.e., laparoscopic cholecystectomy in gallstone pancreatitis), or the patient continues to deteriorate despite maximal supportive care.

▶ **Chronic pancreatitis** - surgery is indicated after medical management has failed and the patient has intractable, severe pain. If the pancreatic duct is > 6 mm in diameter, the patient should be evaluated for a longitudinal pancreaticojejunostomy (Puestow procedure). If the pancreatic duct is < 6 mm, the patient should be evaluated for resection (distal resection, near-total distal resection, pancreaticoduodenectomy, or pancreatic head resection). Nerve blocks and ablation procedures are only minimally effective in treating pain. Conventional pancreatic enzymes are helpful for abd pain, and enteric-coated preparations work well for steatorrhea.

▶ **Pancreatic pseudocyst** - many pseudocysts will spontaneously resolve; surgery is indicated for patients whose symptoms are persistent, in whom the pseudocyst enlarges, or those where pseudocyst develops complications. Surgical options include percutaneous drainage, endoscopic drainage, laparotomy with internal drainage, or laparoscopic internal drainage. Endoscopic treatment: (1) transpapillary approach can be used if cyst does not communicate with the pancreatic duct or (2) transmural approach if cyst < 10 cm, visible bulge, and no vessels.

▶ **Pancreatic cancer** - resection is the only possible cure; only those patients without metastatic disease or vascular invasion are candidates for resection. Adjuvant radiation and chemotherapy remain controversial. Preoperative drainage of the obstructed biliary tree should not be performed. Coagulopathies should be corrected with vit K and fresh frozen plasma. Patients should be evaluated for a pancreaticoduodenectomy (Whipple procedure), pylorus-preserving pancreaticoduodenectomy, distal pancreatectomy, subtotal pancreatectomy, or total pancreatectomy. Palliative procedures for biliary obstruction include surgical bypass, endoscopic stenting, or transhepatic stenting; the palliative procedure for bowel obstruction is laparoscopic or open gastrojejunostomy.

▶ **Cystic tumors** - mucinous cystic neoplasms and cystadenocarcinoma require surgical resection with tumor-free margin; intraductal papillary mucinous tumors mandate total pancreatectomy.

TABLE 17-3
RANSON CRITERIA FOR ACUTE PANCREATITIS (NEGATIVE PROGNOSTIC FACTORS)

At presentation	Within 48 hours of onset
- age > 55 - WBC > 16,000 - glucose > 200 (in nondiabetic) - LDH[a] > 350 - AST > 250	- age > 55 - WBC > 15,000 - glucose > 180 (in nondiabetic) - BUN > 16; increase in BUN > 5 - calcium < 8 - drop in HCT > 10% - albumin < 3.2 - LDH > 600 - AST or ALT > 200 - base deficit > 4 - PaO$_2$ < 60 - fluid sequestration > 6 L

[a]LDH, lactate dehydrogenase.

REFERENCES

1. Norton JA, Bollinger RR, Chang AE, et al. *Surgery, Basic Science and Clinical Evidence.* New York: Springer-Verlag, 2001.
2. Schwartz SI, Shires GT, Spencer FC, et al. *Principles of Surgery.* New York: McGraw-Hill, 1999.
3. Bland KI. *The Practice of General Surgery.* Philadelphia: WB Saunders, 2002.
4. Townsend CM, Beauchamp RD, Evers BM, et al. *Sabiston Textbook of Surgery: The Biologic Basis of Modern Surgical Practice.* Philadelphia: WB Saunders Company, 2001.
5. Feldman M, Scharschmidt BF, Sleisenger MH. *Sleisenger & Fordtran's Gastrointestinal and Liver Disease.* 6th ed. Philadelphia: WB Saunders, 1998.
6. Yamada Y, editor. *Textbook of Gastroenterology.* 3rd ed. Philadelphia: Lippincott Williams & Wilkins, 1999.
7. Goldman L, Bennett JC, eds. *Cecil Textbook of Medicine.* 21st ed. Philadelphia: WB Saunders, 2000.
8. Baillie J. Pancreas divisum. *Clin Perspect Gastroenterol* 2002;5(2):73–76.
9. Sweeney JT, Ulrich CD. Genetics of pancreatic disease. *Clin Perspect Gastroenterol* 2002;5(2):110–116.
10. Grendell JH. Acute pancreatitis. *Clin Perspect Gastroenterol* 2000;3(6): 327–333.
11. Binmoeller KF. Endoscopic treatment of pseudocysts. *Clin Perspect Gastroenterol* 2000;3(6):334–342.
12. Cello JP. Octreotide. *Clin Perspect Gastroenterol* 2000;3(6):349–352.
13. Hawes RH. A clinician's perspective on chronic pancreatitis—2002. *Rev Gastroenterol Dis* 2002;2(2):57–65.
14. Frandzel S. Patient profile highly predictive of post-ERCP pancreatitis. *Gastroenterol Endoscop News* 2001;52(8):12–13.
15. Yoder A. Nutrition support in pancreatitis: beyond parenteral nutrition. *Pract Gastroenterol* 2003;XXVII(1):19–30.

PART IV

MULTISYSTEM DISORDERS

CHAPTER 18

ENDOCRINE SYNDROMES

ENDOCRINE SYNDROMES
Highlights

▶ **Helpful in Differentiating Syndromes:**
- location of tumor
- symptoms and demographics
- lab profile
- imaging studies

▶ **Major Syndromes:**
- insulinoma
- gastrinoma (Zollinger-Ellison syndrome, ZES)
- VIPoma (Verner-Morrison syndrome)
- glucagonoma
- somatostatinoma
- GRFoma (growth hormone-releasing factor)
- carcinoid syndrome
- MEN-I (multiple endocrine neoplasia)

▶ nonfunctional > functional tumors

▶ carcinoid → insulinoma = gastrinoma → all others

▶ OctreoScan - can help distinguish neuroendocrine tumors from other mass lesions and able to stage disease at same time

Demographics

▶ **Insulinoma** - most common symptomatic tumor of the pancreas; 70–80% of the solitary tumors of the pancreas; 5–10% malignant

- **Gastrinoma** - 85% located within gastrinoma triangle (cystic duct, 3rd portion of duodenum, isthmus of pancreas), 30–40% of tumors in duodenal mucosa and 60–80% in pancreas, 50–60% malignant, 50% multiple lesions, 25% associated with MEN-I, seen in 0.1% of DU patients
- **VIPoma** (vasoactive intestinal peptide) - most often found in pancreas (> 90%), usually large (~ 5 cm), 50% malignant
- **Glucagonoma** - majority in body and tail of pancreas, large (> 5 cm), 50–80% malignant
- **Somatostatinoma** - body of pancreas (56%), small bowel (44%), typically large (> 5 cm); > 70% malignant
- **GRFoma** - 40% associated with ZES, 30% associated with MEN-I; frequently large (> 5 cm), > 60% malignant
- **Carcinoid syndrome** - most common site is appendix and usually nonfunctional, most common location for functional tumor is terminal ileum; small bowel tumors usually not symptomatic until liver mets present; tumors in stomach/esophagus/lung commonly functional; rectal highly malignant and have early mets, however, if < 1 cm, endoscopic treatment curative
- **MEN-I** - autosomal dominant; gene abnormality on chromosome 11q; seen in 25% of gastrinoma patients, 40% of somatostatinoma patients, 33% of GRFoma patients; PPomas and nonfunctional tumors specifically associated with MEN-I: gastrinoma 50%, insulinoma 40%, glucagonoma and VIPoma 5%; 3 P's: pituitary adenoma (60%), hyperparathyroidism (95%), enteropancreatic neuroendocrine tumor (65%), most commonly gastrinoma > insulinoma; genetic defect in long arm of chromosome 11(11q11-q13); multifocal tumors

Symptoms/Signs/Labs

- **Insulinoma** - sx due to hypoglycemia and frequently associated with fasting - mild personality changes, confusion, drowsiness, visual disturbance, coma; also, diaphoresis, pallor, tachycardia
- **Gastrinoma** - due to gastric hypersecretory state; most common sx include hypergastrinemia associated with peptic ulcer diathesis (> 90%) - majority in duodenal bulb, diarrhea (30–40%), and esophagitis (50–60%)

TABLE 18-1
PANCREATIC ENDOCRINE TUMORS

Syndrome	Hormone(s) produced	Primary hormone effects	Pathologic features	Clinical features
Zollinger-Ellison	Gastrin	Gastric acid hypersecretion with basal acid outputs usually > 15 mmol/h (> 15 mEq/h)	Delta cell islet tumors; 10% aberrant (duodenal); 60% malignant	Severe peptic ulcer disease often refractory to therapy; ectopic ulcers; diarrhea; multiple endocrine adenomas (parathyroid, pituitary, adrenal, thyroid)
Insulinoma	Insulin	Hypoglycemia with inappropriately increased serum insulin levels	Beta cell islet tumors; 80–90% benign	Hypoglycemic symptoms
Glucagonoma	Glucagon; pancreatic polypeptide	Hyperglucagonemia → glucose intolerance	Alpha cell islet tumors; 60% malignant	Slow-growing pancreatic tumor; hyperglycemia; eczematoid dermatitis, or necrolytic erythema weight loss; anemia; gastric and intestinal motor abnormalities
Somatostatinoma	Somatostatin; pancreatic polypeptide	Somatostatin inhibits insulin, gastrin, and pancreatic enzyme secretion; decreased bile flow	Delta cell islet tumor	Pancreatic tumor; diarrhea; steatorrhea; gallstones; diabetes mellitus; anemia
Pancreatic cholera	Vasoactive intestinal peptide ? Gastric inhibitory polypeptide ? Prostaglandin E ? Pancreatic peptide	Net secretion of salt and water by gut	? Delta cell tumor; >50% malignant	Pancreatic tumor with severe watery diarrhea; flushing; weight loss; hypokalemia; hypercalcemia; hypochlorhydria; hyperglycemia; inordinate fecal water and electrolyte losses
Carcinoid	Serotonin; prostaglandins	Altered gut motility; diarrhea	Enterochromaffin cells; non-beta-cell islet tumors	Carcinoid syndrome with flushing; wheezing; diarrhea; alcohol intolerance; hepatomegaly

- ▶ **VIPoma** - due to excessive release of *v*asoactive *i*ntestinal *p*eptide; WDHA syndrome - profuse (1–6 L/day) *w*atery *d*iarrhea (100%), *h*ypokalemia (90–100%), *a*chlorhydria (70%); also dehydration, hyperglycemia (25–50%), hypercalcemia (25%), flushing (20%); also see hypomagnesemia, hypophosphatemia
- ▶ **Glucagonoma** - due to excessive release of glucagon; *triad*: rash + diabetes + weight loss; migratory necrolytic erythema (70–85%) - most characteristic feature, progresses over 7–14 days, occurs most commonly in areas of friction as well as face and distal extremities; glucose intolerance of diabetes (85%), hypoaminoacidemia (80–90%), weight loss (85%), anemia (85%), diarrhea (15%), thromboembolic phenomenon (20%), glossitis (15%)
- ▶ **Somatostatinoma** - due to excessive release of somatostatin; if pancreatic tumor - triad of gallstones (95%), diabetes (95%), and diarrhea (92%); also steatorrhea (80%), hypochlorhydria (85%), weight loss (90%); if intestinal tumor - weight loss (70%), gallbladder disease (40%), diarrhea (38%), diabetes (20%), hypochlorhydria (17%), steatorrhea (12%); association with von Hippel-Lindau syndrome and von Recklinghausen disease
- ▶ **GRFoma** - acromegaly: large extremities, coarsening of facial features, oily skin, malodorous perspiration, hypertrichosis, voice changes, visceral hypertrophy, glucose intolerance
- ▶ **Carcinoid syndrome** - diarrhea (75%), flushing (65%); also SBO, valvular heart disease, endomyo-cardial fibrosis, asthma, pellagra, bronchospasm in 10%

Diagnosis

- ▶ **Insulinoma** - requires documentation of hypoglycemia (glucose < 40 mg/dL) which is associated with an inappropriate increase in plasma insulin – 72-hour fast, positive if serum insulin levels are stable or increase during hypoglycemia or the insulin to glucose ratio is > 0.3 or corrected insulin to glucose ratio is > 0.5
- ▶ **Gastrinoma** - gastrin > 150 pg/mL, basal acid output > 15 mmol/hour, secretin test > 200 pg/mL increase in gastrin
- ▶ **VIPoma** - secretory diarrhea (> 700 mL/day) which is isotonic and persists during fasting + elevated VIP level (normal = 0–170 pg/mL); usually detectable on U/S or CT
- ▶ **Glucagonoma** - elevated plasma glucagon level ≥ 500 pg/mL (normal = 0–150 pg/mL) + appropriate clinical scenario; usually detectable on U/S or CT

► **Somatostatinoma** - elevated somatostatin level + clinical scenario; usually detectable on U/S or CT
► **GRFoma** - elevated growth hormone-releasing factor level + clinical scenario; usually detectable on U/S or CT
► **Carcinoid syndrome** - midgut: elevated 5-hydroxyindoleacetic (5-HIAA) (can get false positives with walnuts, bananas, avocados, Tylenol); foregut: elevated 5-hydroxytryptophan; OctreoScan.

Treatment

► **Insulinoma** - (1) surgery curative in 75–90%; (2) diazoxide drug of choice (150–800 mg/day) with 60% response rate for patients awaiting surgery or those with metastatic disease
► **Gastrinoma** - (1) surgery when possible; (2) PPIs, especially omeprazole with goal of BAO < 10 mEq/hour in nonoperated patients and < 5 mEq/hour in operated patients or those with esophagitis
► **VIPoma** - (1) electrolytes + fluid; (2) octreotide (> 80% response rate)
► **Glucagonoma** - (1) correction of hypoaminoacidemia; (2) octreotide (> 75% response rate)
► **Somatostatinoma** - octreotide
► **GRFoma** - surgical resection if no metastatic disease; otherwise, octreotide
► **Carcinoid syndrome:**
  • metastatic disease → octreotide
  • appendiceal → appendectomy
  • rectal → endoscopic tx if < 1 cm; resection if > 1 cm
  • small bowel → partial resection due to multicentric lesion in 30–50%

REFERENCES

1. Pelley RJ. Gastrointestinal neuroendocrine tumors: rare causes of chronic diarrhea. *Pract Gastroenterol* 2001; XXV(11):37–43.
2. Cello JP. Octreotide. *Clin Perspect Gastroenterol* 2000;3(6):349–352.
3. Yamada Y, ed. *Handbook of Gastroenterology.* Philadelphia: Lippincott Williams & Wilkins, 1998.
4. McNally PR. *GI/Liver Secrets.* 2nd ed. Philadelphia: Hanley & Belfus, 2001.
5. Yamada Y, ed. *Textbook of Gastroenterology.* 3rd ed. Philadelphia: Lippincott Williams & Wilkins, 1999.

CHAPTER 19

PREGNANCY SYNDROMES

PREGNANCY SYNDROMES
Highlights

▶ **Helpful in Differentiating Syndromes:**
  • trimester of pregnancy
  • symptoms and demographics
  • lab profile

▶ **Major Syndromes:**
  • hyperemesis gravidarum
  • intrahepatic cholestasis of pregnancy
  • HELLP (*h*emolysis, *e*levated *li*ver tests, and *l*ow *p*latelets) syndrome
  • AFLP (acute fatty liver of pregnancy)

Demographics

▶ **Hyperemesis gravidarum** - 1st trimester (rare after 20 weeks), 0.3–0.8% of pregnancies, may recur sporadically during pregnancy and in subsequent pregnancy

▶ **Intrahepatic cholestasis of pregnancy** - 2nd trimester, at risk for recurrence with subsequent pregnancies (60%); ? linked to MDR3 mutation; most common liver disease unique to pregnancy, more common in Chile and Scandinavia

▶ **HELLP** - 3rd trimester (usually dx'd at 32–34 weeks with range 22–40 weeks), 0.17–0.85% of live births; increased risk (25%) of recurrence with subsequent pregnancies; increased risk of HELLP in patients with gestational thrombocytopenia; 8% of uncomplicated pregnancies; 4–19% of patients with preeclampsia; 1/3 of cases occur postpartum; perinatal mortality up to 35–60%

TABLE 19-1
FACTORS ASSOCIATED WITH HYPEREMESIS GRAVIDARUM[a]

Factor	Odds ratio
Maternal age > 35 y	0.6
High body weight	1.4
Nulliparity	1.4
Cigarette smoker	0.7
Twin gestation	1.5
Fetal loss	.07

[a]Reproduced with permission from Abell T, Riely CA. Hyperemesis gravidarum. *Gastroenterol Clin North Am* 1992;21:836. Klebanoff MA, et al. Epidemiology of vomiting in early pregnancy. *Obstet Gynecol* 66;612:1985.

▶ **AFLP** - 3rd trimester, 1:13K–1:16K deliveries, linked to long chain 3-hydroxyacyl-CoA dehydrogenase (LCHAD) deficiency - autosomal recessive so risk of recurrence is 25% of subsequent pregnancies but rare; most frequent in primigravidas (70%), avg age at onset = 27 yo, increased risk with male and twin gestations, maternal mortality rate of 15% and fetal mortality rate up to 49%

TABLE 19-2
CLINICAL FINDINGS IN HELLP SYNDROME

Incidence	~1% of all pregnancies, especially first pregnancies
	~10% of women with preeclampsia
Onset	Third trimester (median-onset, 33 wks)
Symptoms and signs	
Hypertension, proteinuria, and edema	90%+
Headache	50%
Nausea and vomiting	30%
Abdominal pain	50%
Usual laboratory findings	
Thrombocytopenia	95%, early onset
Abnormal morphologic studies of RBCs	Frequent (fragments, schistocytes)
Prothrombin time	Modest increase in 15%
Fibrin degradation products	Increased early
Aminotransferases	5- to 20-fold increase
Alkaline phosphatase	Normal or modest increase (2-fold)
Bilirubin	Low, unless extensive hemolysis and hepatic necrosis occur
Serum creatinine	Mild increase

Symptoms/Signs/Labs

▶ **Hyperemesis gravidarum** - severe N&V; 50% have elevated LFTs (rare for AST/ALT > 1000), mildly elevated bili < 5

▶ **Intrahepatic cholestasis of pregnancy** - severe pruritus (palms, soles; also trunk and extrem) and jaundice (1–4 weeks after development of jaundice) in mother; premature delivery (60%), fetal demise; elevated bile acid (cholylglycine) best test, also elevated bilirubin up to 6, AST and ALT - 3–4× normal, alk phos - up to 4× normal; liver bx - bland cholestasis, bile plugs in zone 3 (central vein region), intact portal tracts

▶ **HELLP** - associated with preeclampsia (HTN, proteinuria, edema), asxtic - abd pain (most common sx; usually RUQ), N&V, HA, renal failure, jaundice in 5% and seizures in severe cases, 3% mortality rate, complications - DIC, placental abruption, renal failure, ascites, pulmonary or cerebral edema, hepatic infarction - abd pain/fever/AST and ALT > 5000; potential hepatic hematoma; AST and ALT elevated up to 6000 and elevation prior to development of complications, plts often < 100K, low haptoglobin, elevated LDH, peripheral blood smear with schistocytes and burr cells; liver bx - fibrin deposition and hemorrhage localized to periportal areas; maternal mortality up to 8% and fetal mortality up to 35%, mortality rate with rupture of hepatic hematoma > 50%

▶ **AFLP** - malaise, fatigue, anorexia, headache, N&V, RUQ pain, polydipsia, fulminant hepatic failure, preeclampsia present in > 50%, 10% maternal and 20% fetal mortality rate, DIC in up to 50%, pancreatitis in up to 30%, severe hypoglycemia in 25–50%; increased LFTs but usually < 300–1000, bili up to 40, leukocytosis, thrombocytopenia; CT and MRI - hypoattenuation of liver; liver bx - microvesicular fat deposits visualized with oil-red O

Treatment

▶ **Hyperemesis gravidarum** - IVF, anti-emetics (promethazine, ondansetron, droperidol)

▶ **Intrahepatic cholestasis of pregnancy** - early delivery at 36–38 weeks, cholestyramine + vit K, UDCA; symptoms usually resolve a few weeks after delivery

▶ **HELLP** - delivery; resolution usually w/in days of delivery, including normal LFTs w/in 3–5 days; plasmapheresis for patients whose plts continue to decrease after delivery

▶ **AFLP** - medical and obstetric emergency: delivery, transfer to center capable of liver transplant if needed; complete recovery may take up to 1 month, but no long-term hepatic sequelae

REFERENCES

1. Feldman M, Scharschmidt BF, Sleisenger MH. *Sleisenger & Fordtran's Gastrointestinal and Liver Disease.* 6th ed. Philadelphia: WB Saunders, 1998.
2. Yamada Y, ed. *Textbook of Gastroenterology.* 3rd ed. Philadelphia: Lippincott Williams & Wilkins, 1999.
3. Cappell MS, guest ed. Gastrointestinal disorders during pregnancy. In: *Gastroenterology Clinics of North America.* Philadelphia: WB Saunders, March 2003.

CHAPTER 20

CLINICAL NUTRITION

CLINICAL NUTRITION
Topics Summary

1. basic principles of nutrient absorption
2. nutrition assessment
3. enteral and parenteral nutrition: basic principles
4. disease-specific nutrition for selected GI diseases
5. ethical considerations in nutrition support

1. Basic Principles of Nutrient Absorption: Highlights

► lipid absorption
► carbohydrate absorption
► protein absorption
► absorption of selected micronutrients - iron, calcium, vit B_{12}, folic acid

Lipid Absorption: General Information

► majority of dietary lipids consumed as *long-chain triglycerides* (LCTs; composed of glycerol and fatty acids more than 12 carbons in length); most lipid in the diet absorbed in upper $2/3$ of the jejunum and must be emulsified prior to absorption; emulsion achieved by chewing of dietary fat and gastric "milling"
► emulsion stabilized when fat droplets are coated by phospholipids; hydrolysis of dietary triglyceride to fatty acids and monoglycerides occurs via pancreatic lipase in the presence of co-lipase
► Bile salts are emulsifying agents and form micelles (disk-shaped structures with the hydrophobic, lipid-soluble portion of the bile salt molecule directed internally and the hydrophilic water-soluble portion directed externally).

▶ Lipid is delivered to brush border membrane of the enterocyte via micelles and other lipid-containing particles.

▶ Most lipids move across this membrane via passive diffusion.

▶ Triglyceride is re-synthesized in the enterocyte and its esters and phospholipids are assembled, along with cholesterol, primarily into chylomicrons during the fed state and into very low density lipoproteins (VLDLs) during the fasted state.

▶ Apolipoprotein B (apo B) is an apoprotein forming a portion of the surface of the chylomicron and is essential for the synthesis and secretion of chylomicrons.

▶ Chylomicrons are secreted into the lymphatic circulation and enter the systemic circulation via the thoracic duct.

Lipid Absorption: Clinical Pearls

▶ *Medium-chain triglycerides* (MCTs; triglycerides composed of glycerol backbone and fatty acids with 6–12 carbons) can be used as a source of fat calories in patients with certain small bowel diseases and in pancreatic exocrine insufficiency.

▶ They can be absorbed in the absence of pancreatic enzymes and do not require re-assembly by the enterocyte into chylomicrons.

▶ MCTs are more water soluble than LCTs and can be transported directly to the liver in the portal venous circulation.

▶ Abetalipoproteinemia is the congenital absence of apo B and results in an inability to produce and secrete chylomicrons; malabsorption of fat and fat-soluble vitamins occurs.

▶ Steatorrhea in Zollinger-Ellison syndrome (ZES) can occur because of reduced luminal pH in the duodenum with resultant inactivation of pancreatic lipase, precipitation of bile acids, and reduced solubility of fatty acids in micelles.

Carbohydrate Absorption: General Information

▶ Dietary sources of carbohydrate include starch (comprised of long chains of glucose molecules), sugars including lactose, fructose, glucose, and sucrose), and fiber (dietary carbohydrates that cannot be hydrolyzed by intestinal or pancreatic enzymes).

▶ Dietary fiber is partially broken down by colonic bacterial enzymes to produce short-chain fatty acids which are used as oxidative fuels by the colonocytes.

► Carbohydrate digestion is initiated by salivary amylase.
► Pancreatic amylase is the major enzyme involved in starch digestion, acting on starch and producing oligosaccharides, maltotriose, maltose, and alpha-limit dextrins; these products, along with sucrose and lactose must be hydrolyzed by brush border enzymes (which include lactase, maltase, alpha-limit dextrinase, sucrase, isomaltase, and trehalase) in order to be absorbed.
► The three major monosaccharides in the diet are glucose, galactose, and fructose and are absorbed via carrier-mediated transport systems in the enterocyte brush border membrane.
► A sodium-glucose co-transporter exists in the brush border membrane; glucose can enhance the absorption of sodium via an active carrier and subsequently water absorption can occur via solvent drag.
► These sugars exit the cell via the basolateral membrane to the interstitial space and diffuse into the portal circulation.

Carbohydrate Absorption: Clinical Pearls
► Oral rehydration therapy exploits the sodium-glucose transporter in the brush border membrane; the presence of glucose in the small bowel lumen enhances sodium absorption and results in water absorption via solvent drag.
► This mechanism of sodium and water absorption often remains intact in diarrheal illnesses including cholera; oral rehydration solutions (i.e., Pedialyte, World Health Organization glucose-based solution, etc.) containing carbohydrate, sodium, potassium, chloride, and base (bicarbonate or citrate) in appropriate proportions can be used to treat diarrhea, short bowel syndrome, and high-output ostomies.

Protein Absorption: General Information
► protein digestion initiated via pepsins secreted by gastric mucosa
► pancreatic proteases (trypsin, chymotrypsin, elastase, carboxypeptidase A and B) all secreted as proenzymes
► Enterokinase or enteropeptidase, an enzyme in the brush border, released from the brush border by bile acids, acts to convert trypsinogen into trypsin.
► Trypsin subsequently activates the pancreatic proteases and continues to convert trypsinogen into trypsin. After the action

of pancreatic proteases, 30% of the amino nitrogen in the lumen is in the form of amino acids, and 70% is in the form of oligopeptides (two to six amino acids in length).

► Amino acids are absorbed as monomers or as di- or tripeptides.

► Peptidases found in the brush border and cytoplasm hydrolyze oligopeptides up to eight amino acids long.

► Multiple transporter systems exist for small peptides and single amino acids.

► Amino acids exit the enterocyte via the basolateral membrane via active transport and diffusion.

Absorption of Selected Nutrients: General Information

► **Iron absorption** - majority of iron absorbed in proximal small bowel; ferrous iron (Fe^{2+}) converted to ferric iron (Fe^{3+}) prior to absorption; Fe^{3+} is not soluble at a pH > 3; gastric acid, some sugars, and amino acids can enhance absorption, and oxalate, phosphate, and phytate can cause precipitation of iron and decrease its absorption.

► **Calcium absorption and the role of Vitiman D** - two major mechanisms of calcium absorption known: (1) active transcellular transport (primarily in the duodenum) and (2) passive paracellular transport (throughout the small bowel); vit D acts to enhance calcium absorption by increasing calcium absorption via the passive paracellular route, which occurs via tight junctions; vitamin D_3 (cholecalciferol) is the major dietary form of vitamin D; most of the vitamin D requirement is produced by endogenous synthesis in the skin during sunlight exposure; concentration of the calcium binding protein in the cytoplasm, called calbindin, is rate-limiting factor in calcium absorption; 1,25-dihydroxyvitamin D regulates calbindin concentration; the liver produces 25-hydroxyvitamin D from vit D and the kidney produces 1,25-dihydroxyvitamin D from 25-hydroxyvitamin D.

► **Vitamin B_{12} absorption** - vit B_{12} (cobalamin) found primarily in animal products, ingested bound to dietary proteins, and released from the proteins by gastric acid; salivary R protein binds to the cobalamin in the stomach; in the duodenum, pancreatic enzymes cleave the R protein and intrinsic factor, produced by gastric parietal cells, binds to cobalamin. The intrinsic factor-cobalamin complex passes into the terminal ileum and binds to receptors in the terminal ileum. The complex is absorbed and transported to the liver via the portal circulation.

▶ **Folic acid absorption** - folate absorption accomplished following hydrolysis at the brush border membrane and incorporation into the cytoplasm; uptake via carrier-mediated mechanism, which is sodium-dependent process active at acid pH; the transport process is inhibited by diphenylhydantoin and sulfasalazine

Absorption of Selected Nutrients: Clinical Pearls

▶ Iron deficiency is a common manifestation of celiac dz. The proximal small intestine is often more severely affected in celiac dz. For this reason, there can be significant malabsorption of nutrients which rely primarily on functional small bowel mucosa for their absorption, such as iron.

▶ Vit B_{12} deficiency can be seen in a variety of GI disorders, including pernicious anemia (lack of intrinsic factor), achlorhydria (suboptimal release of vit B_{12} from dietary proteins), pancreatic insufficiency (defective release of the vitamin from R protein), bacterial overgrowth (consumption of vit B_{12} by bacteria), and diseased or surgically resected ileum (lack of receptors for intrinsic factor-cobalamin complex).

▶ Sulfasalazine can result in folate deficiency by inhibiting carrier-mediated uptake of folate into the enterocyte. Patients on sulfasalazine therapy should also receive folate supplementation.

2. Nutritional Assessment: Highlights

▶ history and physical exam (H&P)
▶ anthropometric measurements
▶ laboratory indices

H&P: General Information

▶ Medical history should include information regarding acute and chronic medical illnesses, surgery, medications, or other therapies with a potential for influencing nutrition, psychosocial history (including socioeconomic status, use of cigarettes and alcohol). Additional useful information includes weight change, appetite, GI symptoms (including nausea, vomiting, change in bowel habits, and stool consistency), diet history (food patterns, eating habits and ability to obtain and prepare food, use of vitamin supplements), dietary restrictions, food allergies/intolerances, and activity level.

▶ Physical examination should emphasize measurement of weight, skin inspection for evidence of poor wound healing, and skin turgor. The oral cavity should be examined for evidence of glossitis and angular stomatitis (both seen in B vitamin deficiency) and the appearance of hair and nails, presence of edema, muscle tone and strength, muscle wasting, fat stores, sensation, and mental status.

Anthropometric Measurements: General Information

▶ Anthropometric measurements provide information regarding lean body mass and fat stores. They include height, weight, body mass index (weight in kg/height in m^2), triceps skinfold measurement (measurement of subcutaneous fat) and mid-arm circumference (measurement of skeletal muscle mass), and bioimpedance analysis (to measure fat-free mass and total body water).

Laboratory Indices: General Information

▶ **Hepatic proteins, including albumin, transferrin, prealbumin, and retinol-binding protein** - *Albumin* is easy and inexpensive to measure and correlates with outcome, length of hospital stay, and risk of complications, but use is limited by its relatively long half-life (14–20 days). Because of long half-life, changes in nutritional status are not immediately reflected by the albumin level. Use is also limited by factors other than nutritional status which may affect the albumin level (i.e., liver disease, hydration status, etc.). *Transferrin* has a shorter half-life and is a more useful index of nutritional status in patients with liver dz. *Pre-albumin* has a shorter half-life than albumin and transferrin (2–3 days), but has a greater sensitivity to non-nutritional factors (infection, bleeding, fever). *Retinol-binding protein* is used least frequently in the clinical setting. It has a 12-hour half-life, but use is limited by acute sensitivity to non-nutritional factors.

▶ **Total lymphocyte count** - a measure of immune function and a reflection of nutritional status; influenced by many factors other than nutritional status and of limited clinical use in measurement of nutritional status

▶ **Delayed hypersensitivity skin testing** - a measure of cell-mediated immunity; influenced by many factors other than nutritional status and of limited clinical use in measurement of nutritional status

3. Basic Enteral and Parenteral Nutrition and Selection of Appropriate Nutritional Regimen

Enteral Nutrition: Highlights
► indications and strategy for patient selection
► contraindications
► advantages of enteral nutrition
► formula categories
► types of enteral access
► risks of enteral nutrition

Enteral Nutrition: General Information
► **Indications** - should be considered in all patients whose oral intake is insufficient to maintain nutritional needs and are expected to be unable to achieve adequate oral intake for > 7 days (or > 5–7 days if malnourished); need functional gut, but even a significant degree of gut pathology does not preclude enteral feedings under all circumstances
► **Contraindications** - high output proximal fistula, severe acute pancreatitis, severe nausea and vomitting or diarrhea, mechanical obstruction, GIB, hemodynamic instability, gut ischemia, bowel obstruction, chronic idiopathic intestinal pseudo-obstruction, GI tract fistula [unless when enteral access can be placed distal to the fistula or fistula output is relatively low (< 200 mL/day)], severe ileus, severe malabsorption (as may occur in massive small bowel resection, radiation enteritis, etc.), inability to provide adequate nutrients and fluid via the enteral route, or inability to obtain enteral access
► **Advantages** (as compared to parenteral nutrition) - lower cost, fewer infectious complications, and maintenance of gut mucosal integrity and function
► **Enteral formulas:**
  • *polymeric formulas*: contain whole proteins, glucose polymers, and lipids as LCTs or a combination of LCTs and MCTs
  • *semi-elemental formulas*: consist of protein in the form of hydrolyzed casein, whey, or lactalbumin and contain small peptides and, in some formulas, free amino acids; carbohydrate present as simple sugars, glucose polymers, or starch;

fat present as LCTs or a combination of LCTs and MCTs; more expensive than standard polymeric formulas and, for most disease states, no clear advantage has been established for their use

- *elemental formulas*: devised because they require minimal gut function for absorption; typically composed of free amino acids, glucose polymers, and minimal fat in form of long-chain fatty acids; in absence of pancreatic insufficiency, absorption of elemental formulas not proven to be better than absorption of semi-elemental and polymeric formulas; no clear benefit established in most disease states

▶ **Types of enteral access**:
- *nasogastric*: for short-term enteral nutrition
- *orogastric*: short-term enteral nutrition in mechanically ventilated patients
- *surgical or percutaneous endoscopic gastrostomy* (PEG): for enteral nutrition patients requiring enteral feedings > 4–6 weeks
- *naso- or oro-duodenal:* for short-term enteral nutrition in patients intolerant of gastric feedings
- *naso- or oro-jejunal*: short-term feeding for patients requiring feedings distal to the ligament of Treitz
- *percutaneous endoscopic gastrostomy with jejunal extension* (PEGJ): for long-term enteral feedings, especially in patients who require jejunal feedings with concurrent gastric suction
- *surgical or direct percutaneous endoscopic gastrostomy*: for those requiring long-term jejunal feedings

▶ **Risks of enteral feeding** - improper placement of feeding tubes (including tracheal or bronchial intubation), metabolic complications such as electrolyte and glucose disturbances (most commonly hyponatremia, hypokalemia, hypophosphatemia, and hyperglycemia). Care must be taken to prevent re-feeding syndrome (a group of metabolic and physiologic disturbances which can occur when re-feeding severely malnourished patients). Patients at risk include those with prolonged npo status (> 7–10 days), anorexia nervosa, chronic malnutrition, chronic alcoholism, morbid obesity with significant weight loss, etc. Consequences of this syndrome include a rise in serum insulin with subsequent intracellular movement of electrolytes and a drop in serum magnesium, potassium, and phosphorus. The rise in serum insulin prevents glycogenolysis, and gluconeogenesis and low-serum glucose can occur. CHF, arrhythmia, and respiratory failure can occur. Correction of electrolytes before initiation of feeding, slow advancement of feedings with close clinical monitoring for hypokalemia, hypomagnesemia and hypophosphatemia, and monitoring for the development of CHF and respiratory decompensation are all critical.

Parenteral Nutrition: Highlights
▶ indications
▶ contraindications
▶ content of parenteral nutrition
▶ risks of parenteral nutrition

Parenteral Nutrition: General Information
▶ **Indications** - a condition that precludes use of the GI tract for 1 week or more; in critically ill patients, when the gut cannot be used and a hypermetabolic state is anticipated for > 4–5 days
▶ **Contraindications** - metabolic disturbances such as severe hyperglycemia, azotemia, encephalopathy and hyperosmolality, and severe derangements in electrolyte levels or fluid balance, inability to obtain venous access, or a medical condition with a poor prognosis for which aggressive nutrition support would be inappropriate
▶ **Components of parenteral nutrition** - (1) *carbohydrate* generally in the form of *dextrose; glycerol or glycerin* occasionally used in some peripherally administered solutions to minimize vascular irritation; (2) *protein* administered in the form of *amino acids.* (Specialty amino acid formulations have been devised for use in patients with renal failure and hepatic insufficiency. Renal formulations contain primarily essential amino acids. The rationale is nonessential amino acids can be recycled from urea, but essential amino acids must be provided in the diet. Hepatic formulas have increased quantities of branched-chain amino acids based on the theory that a lower ratio of aromatic to branched-chain amino acids will decrease the formation of false neurotransmitters thought to have an adverse effect in hepatic encephalopathy. These formulations are more expensive and have not been found to have significant clinical benefit in renal

or hepatic disease. Other modified amino acid preparations containing increased amounts of branched-chain amino acids are available for use in patients with hypermetabolism, burns, trauma, or metabolic stress. They do not have any proven positive impact on outcome); (3) *lipid emulsions* in the form of *long-chain triglycerides*; additional components include *electrolytes, minerals, vitamins, and trace elements.*

▶ **Types of parenteral nutrition:**
  - Peripheral parenteral nutrition (PPN) has lower dextrose concentrations (5–10%) and amino acid concentrations (3%) than centrally administered total parenteral nutrition (TPN). It is indicated when mild to moderate malnutrition exists in patients who cannot be fed orally or enterally or when central vein parenteral administration is not feasible and is typically used for 2 weeks or less due to irritation of peripheral veins and limited patient tolerance.
  - TPN has a glucose content of 15–25% and can provide all of a patient's nutritional needs. It must be administered via a central vein (usually superior vena cava) to prevent venous irritation.

▶ **Complications** - catheter-related complications, including trauma related to insertion (pneumothorax, arterial injury, air embolism, catheter thrombosis) and sepsis, metabolic complications, and hepatobiliary complications (e.g., elevated transaminases and alkaline phosphatase, steatosis, steatohepatitis, cirrhosis, acalculous cholecystitis, formation of gallbladder sludge, and cholelithiasis)

4. Disease-Specific Nutrition for Selected Gastrointestinal Conditions: Highlights

▶ nutrition support in pancreatitis
▶ nutrition support in Crohn's disease
▶ nutrition support in hepatic disease
▶ nutrition support in short bowel syndrome

Nutrition Support in Pancreatitis: General Information

▶ Mild to moderate acute pancreatitis generally results in resumption of an oral diet within 7 days. Specialized nutrition support may not be required. When nutrition support is required (i.e., slow resolution of mild to moderate pancreatitis), enteral feedings into the jejunum distal to the ligament of Treitz are safe, efficacious, less costly, and associated with less risk than parenteral nutrition. This type of feeding is associated with less pancreatic exocrine secretion because of elimination of cephalic and gastric phases of pancreatic secretion.

▶ Parenteral nutrition is recommended in patients with severe pancreatitis and should be initiated within the first 72 hours of admission.

▶ In chronic pancreatitis a high-calorie, high-protein diet with moderate fat and carbohydrate is recommended. Use of pancreatic enzymes is recommended to treat maldigestion.

▶ Energy needs in chronic pancreatitis fall in the range of 30–35 kcals/kg/day. If steatorrhea cannot be adequately controlled with pancreatic enzymes, dietary fat should be reduced. Supplementation with fat-soluble vitamins should be provided.

Nutrition Support in Crohn's Disease: General Information

▶ Patients with milder Crohn's disease can often maintain oral feedings. In more severe Crohn's disease, parenteral nutrition can be useful in facilitating closure of fistulas which cannot be managed with enteral feedings. It can also be used to correct malnutrition in the preoperative setting. Both enteral and parenteral nutrition can be used to treat growth failure in children and can result in remission, but symptoms may recur with re-institution of oral diet.

Nutrition Support in Hepatic Disease: General Information

▶ Fulminant hepatitis should be initially managed with 10% dextrose infusion to prevent hypoglycemia. If no contraindications exist, enteral feedings can be given. If ileus is present, parenteral nutrition can be given with 0.6 g/kg/day of standard amino acids with about 30–35 kcals/kg/day administered with a mixture of carbohydrates and lipids. Patients with negative nitrogen balance and severe hepatic encephalopathy can be given parenteral nutrition with branched chain amino acids. Fluids and sodium should be restricted as needed to control intracranial pressure and resume normal protein intake when condition improves.

▶ In compensated cirrhosis, a diet with normal protein, high-complex carbohydrates, and 30–35 kcals/kg/day is recommended with 1.2 g/kg/day of protein. Frequent small meals with a bedtime snack are recommended. Multivitamins and calcium, zinc, and magnesium supplements are advised, with water and sodium restriction only when clinically indicated.

► Protein restriction is indicated in the setting of hepatic encephalopathy (0.6–0.8 g/kg/day), but restriction should be temporary in the setting of acute encephalopathy until the cause of encephalopathy is uncovered.

► Enteral feedings with 35 kcals/kg/day can improve LFTs and shorten the hospital stay in acute alcoholic hepatitis. Normal quantities of protein (1–1.2 kcals/kg) should be given.

Nutrition Support in Short Bowel Syndrome:
General Information

► Short bowel syndrome is the syndrome resulting from extensive small bowel resection.

► Patients with an intact colon and ileocecal valve tolerate small bowel resection with fewer adverse effects because of enhanced water and sodium absorption. The colon can also recover energy from malabsorbed carbohydrates by bacterial fermentation of carbohydrates to short-chain fatty acids which are absorbed. Intestinal adaptation continues for 1–3 years postresection.

► During the initial post-op period, parenteral nutrition is required. During the next phase, a low-osmolality diet or introduction of an isotonic enteral formula is indicated. H2 blockers or PPIs should be given to decrease the gastric acid hypersecretion that occurs in these patients and results in peptic disease and increased volume of diarrhea when untreated.

► Drugs to reduce intestinal motility (such as loperamide, diphenoxylate, or tincture of opium) should be used to reduce stool output. Octreotide can also reduce stool volume.

► Oral rehydration solutions given in a volume of 1–3 L/day can often preclude the need for parenteral hydration.

5. Ethical Considerations in Nutritional Support

► Primary concerns include the initiation and termination of nutrition support.

► Decisions regarding initiation and termination of feeding should take into consideration the underlying disease state, and a patient's personal beliefs and wishes.

► The decision to place a PEG in patients with end-stage malignancy and advanced dementia should be carefully considered. The shortest post-PEG survival is seen in these patients, with

30-day mortality rates in the 22–24% range, reflecting the high mortality of the underlying disease entity.

▶ Court decisions have determined that artificial nutrition, like other therapeutic interventions, can be withheld, initiated, or withdrawn depending upon a patient's clinical condition.

▶ Enteral and parenteral nutrition may be contraindicated in patients who are not candidates for aggressive therapy because of the severity of underlying disease or the patient's personal wishes.

▶ Patients have the right to accept or decline artificial nutrition. Care should be taken to assure that the potential benefits, risks, and ramifications of the initiation and termination of artificial nutrition are fully understood by the patient and family, or surrogate.

REFERENCES

1. Marsh MN, Riley SA. Digestion and absorption of nutrients and vitamins. In: Feldman M, Scharschmidt BF, Sleisenger M, eds. *Gastrointestinal and Liver Disease*. 6th ed. Philadelphia: WB Saunders, 1998:1471-1500.
2. Klein S, Fleming CR. Enteral and Parenteral Nutrition. In: Feldman M, Scharschmidt BF, Slesinger M, eds. *Gastrointestinal and Liver Disease*. 6th ed. Phildelphia: WB Saunders, 1998:254-277.
3. Gottschlich MA, Fuhrman MP, Hammond KA, et al. *The Science Practice of Nutrition Support: A Case Based Core Curriculum*. Dubuque, IA: Kendall/Hunt Publishing Co, 2001.
4. Yoder AJ. Nutrition support in pancreatitis: beyond parenteral nutrition. *Pract Gastroenterol* 2003;27:19-30.
5. Nightengale JMD. Management of patients with a short bowel. *Nutrition* 1999;15:633-637.
6. DiSario JA, Baskin WN, Brown RD, et al. Endoscopic approaches to enteral nutrition support. *Gastrointest Endoscop* 2002;55:901-908.
7. Huang ZB, Ahronheim JC. Nutrition and hydration in terminally ill patients: an update. *Clin Geriatr Med* 2000;16:313-325.
8. Lipman TO. Enteral Nutrition and Dying: Ethical Issues in the Termination of Enteral Nutrition in Adults. In: Rombeau JL, Rolandelli RH, eds. *Clinical Nutrition: Enteral and Tube Feeding*. 3rd ed. Philadelphia: WB Saunders, 1996;588-598.

CHAPTER 21

NUTRITIONAL/VITAMIN DEFICIENCY AND TOXICITY SYNDROMES

NUTRITIONAL/VITAMIN DEFICIENCY AND TOXICITY SYNDROMES

Highlights

► **Helpful in Differentiating Syndromes:**
  - sources and absorption
  - symptoms and demographics
  - lab profile

► **Major Deficiency Syndromes:**
  - vit A (retinol)
  - vit E (tocopherol)
  - vit K
  - thiamine (B_1)
  - riboflavin (B_2)
  - niacin (nicotinic acid; B_3)
  - pyridoxine (B_6)
  - cobalamin (B_{12})
  - folate (folic acid)
  - ascorbic acid (vitamin C)
  - zinc
  - copper
  - selenium
  - chromium
  - manganese
  - molybdenum

► **Major Toxicity Syndromes:**
  - vit A (retinol)
  - vit E (tocopherol)

TABLE 21-1
RECOMMENDED DIETARY ALLOWANCES

Category	Age, years, or condition	Weight[b] kg	lb	Height[b] cm	in	Protein, g	Vit A, μg RE[c]	Vit E, mg α-TE[d]	Vit K, μg	Vit C, mg	Iron, mg	Zinc, mg	Iodine, μg	Selenium, μg
Infants	0.0–0.5	6	13	60	24	13	375	3	5	30	6	5	40	10
	0.5–1.0	9	20	71	28	14	375	4	10	35	10	5	50	15
Children	1–3	13	29	90	35	16	400	6	15	40	10	10	70	20
	4–6	20	44	112	44	24	500	7	20	45	10	10	90	20
	7–10	28	62	132	52	28	700	7	30	45	10	10	120	30
Males	11–14	45	99	157	62	45	1000	10	45	50	12	15	150	40
	15–18	66	145	176	69	59	1000	10	65	60	12	15	150	50
	19–24	72	160	177	70	58	1000	10	70	60	10	15	150	70
	25–50	79	174	176	70	63	1000	10	80	60	10	15	150	70
	51+	77	170	173	68	63	1000	10	80	60	10	15	150	70
Females	11–14	46	101	157	62	46	800	8	45	50	15	12	150	45
	15–18	55	120	163	64	44	800	8	55	60	15	12	150	50
	19–24	58	128	164	65	46	800	8	60	60	15	12	150	55
	25–50	63	138	163	64	50	800	8	65	60	15	12	150	55
	51+	65	143	160	63	50	800	8	65	60	10	12	150	55
Pregnant						60	800	10	65	70	30	15	175	65
Lactating	1st 6 mos					65	1300	12	65	95	15	19	200	75
	2nd mos					62	1200	11	65	90	15	16	200	75

[a]This table does not include nutrients for which dietary reference intakes have recently been established. (See *Dietary Reference Intakes for Calcium, Phosphorus, Magnesium, Vitamin D, and Fluoride and Dietary Reference Intakes for Thiamin, Riboflavin, Niacin, Vitamin B$_6$, Folate, Vitamin B$_{12}$, Pantothenic Acid, Biotin, and Choline.* Washington DC: National Academy Press, 1997 and 1998, respectively.) The allowances, expressed as average daily intakes over time, are intended to provide for individual variations among most normal persons as they live in the U.S. under usual environmental stresses. Diets should be based on a variety of common foods in order to provide other nutrients for which human requirements have been less well defined.

[b]Weights and heights of Reference Adults are actual medians for the U.S. population of the designated age. The use of these figures does not imply that the height-to-weight ratios are ideal.

[c]Retinol equivalents. 1 retinol equivalent = 1 μg retinol or 6 μg β-carotene.

[d]α-Tocopherol equivalents. 1 mg d-α tocopherol = 1 α-TE.

Source: Reprinted with permission from Food and Nutrition Board, National Academy of Sciences—National Research Council Recommended Dietary Allowances, Revised 1989 (Abridged). Courtesy of the National Academy Press, Washington, DC.

TABLE 21-2
RECOMMENDED INTAKES FOR INDIVIDUALS[a]

Life-stage group	Calcium, mg/d	Phosphorus, mg/d	Magnesium, mg/d	Vit D, μg/d[b,c]	Fluoride, mg/d	Thiamine, mg/d
Infants						
0–6 mo	210	100	30	5	0.01	0.2
7–12 mo	270	275	75	5	0.5	0.3
Children						
1–3 y	500	**460**	80	5	0.7	**0.5**
4–8 y	800	**500**	130	5	1	**0.6**
Males						
9–13 y	1300	**1250**	240	5	2	**0.9**
14–18 y	1300	**1250**	410	5	3	**1.2**
19–30 y	1000	**700**	400	5	4	**1.2**
31–50 y	1000	**700**	420	5	4	**1.2**
51–70 y	1200	**700**	420	10	4	**1.2**
>70 y	1200	**700**	420	15	4	**1.2**
Females						
9–13 y	1300	**1250**	240	5	2	**0.9**
14–18 y	1300	**1250**	360	5	3	**1.0**
19–30 y	1000	**700**	310	5	3	**1.1**
31–50 y	1000	**700**	320	5	3	**1.1**
51–70 y	1200	**700**	320	10	3	**1.1**
>70 y	1200	**700**	320	15	3	**1.1**
Pregnancy						
≤18 y	1300	**1250**	400	5	3	**1.4**
19–30 y	1000	**700**	350	5	3	**1.4**
31–50 y	1000	**700**	360	5	3	**1.4**
Lactation						
≤18 y	1300	**1250**	360	5	3	**1.5**
19–30 y	1000	**700**	310	5	3	**1.5**
31–50 y	1000	**700**	320	5	3	**1.5**

[a]This table presents recommended dietary allowances (RDAs) in bold type and adequate intakes (AIs) in ordinary type. RDAs and AIs may both be used as goals for individual intake. RDAs are set to meet the needs of almost all (97–98%) individuals in a group. For healthy breast fed infants, the AI is the mean intake. The AI for other life-stage and gender groups is believed to cover needs of all individuals in the group, but lack of data or uncertainty in the data prevent being able to specify with confidence the percentage of individuals covered by this intake.

[b]As cholecalciferol. 1 μg cholecalciferol = 40 IU vit D.

[c]In the absence of adequate exposure to sunlight.

[d]As niacin equivalents (NE). 1 mg of niacin = 60 mg of tryptophan; 0–6 mos = preformed niacin (not NE).

[e]As dietary folate equivalents (DFE). 1 DFE = 1 μg food folate = 0.6 μg of folic acid from fortified food or as a supplement consumed with food = 0.5 μg of a supplement taken on an empty stomach.

TABLE 21-2
RECOMMENDED INTAKES FOR INDIVIDUALS[a] (CONTINUED)

Riboflavin, mg/d	Niacin, mg/d[d]	Vit B_6, mg/d	Folate, µg/d[e]	Vit B_{12}, µg/d	Pantothenic acid, mg/d	Biotin, µg/d	Choline, mg/d[f]
0.3	2	0.1	65	0.4	1.7	5	125
0.4	4	0.3	80	0.5	1.8	6	150
0.5	6	0.5	150	0.9	2	8	200
0.6	8	0.6	200	1.2	3	12	250
0.9	12	1.0	300	1.8	4	20	375
1.3	16	1.3	400	2.4	5	25	550
1.3	16	1.3	400	2.4	5	30	550
1.3	16	1.3	400	2.4	5	30	550
1.3	16	1.7	400	2.4[g]	5	30	550
1.3	16	1.7	400	2.4[g]	5	30	550
0.9	12	1.0	300	1.8	4	20	375
1.0	14	1.2	400[h]	2.4	5	25	400
1.1	14	1.3	400[h]	2.4	5	30	425
1.1	14	1.3	400[h]	2.4	5	30	425
1.1	14	1.5	400	2.4[g]	5	30	425
1.1	14	1.5	400	2.4[g]	5	30	425
1.4	18	1.6	600[i]	2.6	6	30	450
1.4	18	1.9	600[i]	2.6	6	30	450
1.4	18	1.9	600[i]	2.6	6	30	450
1.6	17	2.0	500	2.8	7	35	550
1.6	17	2.0	500	2.8	7	35	550
1.6	17	2.0	500	2.8	7	35	550

[f]Although AIs have been set for choline, there are few data to assess whether a dietary supply of choline is needed at all stages of the life cycle, and it may be that the choline requirement can be met by endogenous synthesis at some of these stages.

[g]Because 10–30% of older people may malabsorb food-bound B_{12}, it is advisable for those > 50 y to meet their RDA mainly by consuming foods fortified with B_{12} or a supplement containing B_{12}.

[h]In view of evidence linking inadequate folate intake with neural tube defects in the fetus it is recommended that all women capable of becoming pregnant consume 400 µg from supplements or fortified foods in addition to intake of food folate from a varied diet.

[i]It is assumed that women will continue consuming 400 µg from supplements or fortified food until their pregnancy is confirmed and they enter prenatal care, which ordinarily occurs after the end of the periconceptional period—the critical time for formation of the neural tube.

Source: Reprinted with permission from Food and Nutrition Board, Institute of Medicine—National Academy of Sciences Dietary Reference Intakes, 1999. Courtesy of the National Academy Press, Washington, DC.

TABLE 21-3
DEFICIENCIES AND TOXICITIES OF METALS

Element	Deficiency	Toxicity

Zinc	Growth retardation, ↓ taste and smell, alopecia, dermatitis, diarrhea, immunologic dysfunction, failure to thrive, gonadal atrophy, impaired spermatogenesis, congenital malformations	General
		  Gastritis, sweating, fever, nausea, vomiting
		Occupational
		  Respiratory distress, pulmonary fibrosis

Copper	Anemia, growth retardation, defective keratinization and pigmentation of hair, hypothermia, degenerative changes in aortic elastin, osteopenia, mental deterioration, scurvy-like changes in skeleton	General Nausea, vomiting, diarrhea, hepatic failure, tremor, mental deterioration, hemolytic anemia, renal dysfunction

Selenium	Cardiomyopathy, congestive heart failure, striated muscle degeneration	General
		  Alopecia, nausea, vomiting, abnormal nails, emotional lability, peripheral neuropathy, lassitude, garlic odor to breath, dermatitis
		Occupational
		  Lung and nasal carcinomas, liver necrosis, pulmonary inflammation

Chromium	Impaired glucose tolerance	Occupational Renal failure, dermatitis, pulmonary cancer
Manganese	Bone demineralization, ataxia, convulsions, anemia	Occupational Encephalitis-like syndrome, Parkinson-like syndrome, psychosis, pneumoconiosis

- vit K
- thiamine (B_1)
- riboflavin (B_2)
- niacin (nicotinic acid; B_3)
- pyridoxine (B_6)
- cobalamin (B_{12})

- folate (folic acid)
- ascorbic acid (vitamin C)
- zinc
- copper
- selenium
- chromium
- manganese
- molybdenum

Sources (S) and Absorption Site (A)

▶ **Vitamin A (retinol)** - S: pigmented vegetables and fruit, liver, enriched dairy products; A: jejunum

▶ **Vitamin E (tocopherol)** - S: vegetable oils

▶ **Vitamin K** - S: green leafy vegetables, colonic bacteria; A: proximal jejunum

▶ **Thiamine (B_1)** - S: yeast, pork, legumes

▶ **Riboflavin (B_2)** - S: eggs, lean meat, milk, broccoli, enriched flour; A: proximal small intestine, enterohepatic circulation

▶ **Niacin (nicotinic acid; B_3)** - S: meats, fish, legumes, grains, nuts; A: intestine

▶ **Pyridoxine (B_6)** - S: animal protein, whole grain cereal; A: jejunum; impaired by isoniazid, penicillamine, hydralazine

▶ **Cobalamin (B_{12})** - S: animal sources only, produced by bacteria which are ingested by animals; A: B_{12} complex hydrolyzed in small intestine bound to intrinsic factor and transported across ileum and stored in liver; absorbed in TI

▶ **Folate (folic acid)** - S: ubiquitous in food; vegetables, legumes, kidney, liver, nuts; A: proximal small bowel; impaired by ETOH, anticonvulsants, cholestyramine, sulfasalazine, methotrexate

▶ **Ascorbic acid (vitamin C)** - S: fruits (especially citrus) and vegetables

▶ **Zinc** - S: meat, fish; A: upper small bowel; impaired by dietary binders and pancreatic insufficiency

▶ **Copper** - A: stomach and small bowel; impaired by zinc, iron, and molybdenum

▶ **Selenium** - A: small bowel

▶ **Chromium** - exists in food as chromium-nicotinic acid complex known as glucose tolerance factor

▶ **Essential fatty acids (linoleic, linolenic, and arachidonic acid)** - S: vegetable oils

► **Short-chain fatty acids (acetate, propionate, butyrate)** - stimulate colonic blood flow, colonic fluid and electrolyte absorption; butyrate preferred fuel for colonocyte

► **Biotin** - S: abundant in food (e.g., liver, soy, beans, yeast, egg yolks, nuts, mushrooms, cauliflower)

► **Vitamin D** - S: fish liver oils, eggs, liver, dairy; A: small bowel

► **Iodine** - A: GI tract

Deficiency Syndromes

► **Vitamin A (retinol)** - poor dark (visual) adaptation, xerophthalmia, dry skin, increased infections, altered taste and smell, increased CSF pressure

► **Vitamin E (tocopherol)** - hemolysis, progressive neurologic syndrome (areflexia, gait disturbance, decreased vibratory and proprioceptive sensation, gaze paresis) deficiency rare but can be seen in abetalipoproteinemia, cystic fibrosis, cirrhosis, malabsorption, biliary obstruction, excessive mineral oil ingestion

► **Vitamin K** - prolonged PT, increased risk of hemorrhage

► **Thiamine (B_1)** - (1) wet beriberi: unresponsive severe lactic acidosis, high-output cardiac failure, hypotension or (2) Wernicke-Korsakoff encephalopathy: mental status changes, nystagmus, ophthalmoplegia, ataxia, coma, death (deficiency seen in alcoholics, malabsorption, severe malnutrition, prolonged fever, chronic hemodialysis)

► **Riboflavin (B_2)** - isolated deficiency uncommon; usually in combination with other vitamin deficiencies; sore throat, glossitis, cheilosis, angular stomatitis, seborrheic dermatitis, normochromic/normocytic anemia, pruritus, photophobia, visual impairment

► **Niacin (nicotinic acid; B_3)** pellagra: 4 D's - *d*ermatitis, *d*ementia, *d*iarrhea, *d*eath; angular stomatitis, painful tongue (deficiency seen rarely as complication in alcoholism, malabsorption, carcinoid, Hartnup disease)

► **Pyridoxine (B_6)** - isolated deficiency uncommon; usually in combination with other vit B deficiencies; peripheral neuropathy, seborrheic dermatitis, glossitis, angular stomatitis, cheilosis, seizure, sideroblastic anemia (deficiency seen in alcoholics and malabsorption)

► **Cobalamin (B_{12})** - macrocytic anemia, loss of taste, glossitis, diarrhea, dyspepsia, hair loss, impotence, *neuro* - peripheral neuropathy, loss of vibratory sensation, incoordination, muscle weakness and atrophy, irritability, memory loss; deficiency caused by hypochlorhydria (found in 5–15% of population > 65 yo), pernicious anemia if intrinsic factor deficiency, pancreatic insufficiency, partial/gastric resection, PPIs, bacterial overgrowth, ileal dz

▶ **Folate (folic acid)** - neural tube defects in fetus, megaloblastic anemia, thrombocytopenia, leukopenia, glossitis, diarrhea, fatigue; homocystinemia - may induce/aggravate occlusive vascular dz and colon ca

▶ **Ascorbic acid (vitamin C)** - scurvy: petechiae, perifollicular hemorrhage, inflamed and bleeding gums, edema, impaired wound healing, lethargy; develops after 2–3 months of dietary deficiency; deficiency also caused by alcoholism, malabsorption, Crohn's disease

▶ **Zinc** *dermatologic*: symmetrical involvement of face, scalp, perianal area, hands/feet (pustular, vesicular, bullous, seborrheic, acneiform), alopecia; *neurologic:* personality changes, lethargy, irritability; *other*: growth retardation, dysgeusia, anorexia, male infertility, impaired T-cell function, night blindness; deficiency seen in malabsorption, cirrhosis, alcoholism, nephrotic syndrome, sickle cell anemia, pregnancy, pica, pancreatic insufficiency, chronic diarrhea; low zinc levels with low albumin

▶ **Copper** - dietary deficiency rare: deficiencies seen in parenteral nutrition; neutropenia, hypochromic-microcytic anemia, failure of elastin and collagen cross-linking resulting in vascular rupture, emphysema, and osteoporosis; neurologic disorders, impaired immune function

▶ **Selenium** - (1) Keshan's disease: cardiomyopathy, age 1–9; low soil selenium areas of China; low blood and hair levels in Keshan district of China and (2) PPN/TPN: cardiomyopathy, proximal muscle weakness and/or painful myalgias, RBC macrocytosis, pseudoalbinism; deficiency seen in malabsorption, fistulas, alcoholism, cirrhosis, AIDS, cancer

▶ **Chromium** - hyperglycemia, peripheral neuropathy, encephalopathy, weight loss; deficiency seen in short bowel syndrome

▶ **Manganese** - abnormal glucose intolerance, bone demineralization, ataxia, seizures, anemia

▶ **Molybdenum** - single case report: hypermethionemia, hypouricemia, hypouricosuria, low urinary excretion of sulfate

- ▶ **Essential fatty acids (linoleic, linolenic, and arachidonic acid)** - usually caused by fat-free TPN and appears within 3–6 weeks; dermatitis: dry, scaly skin progressing to exfoliative dermatitis; alopecia, coarse hair, hepatomegaly, thrombocytopenia, diarrhea, growth retardation
- ▶ **Biotin** - anorexia, nausea, dermatitis, alopecia, depression, organic aciduria; deficiency seen in diets high in egg whites, PPN/TPN deficient in biotin
- ▶ **Vitamin D** - hypocalcemia, hypophosphatemia, bone demineralization, osteomalacia in adults, rickets in children, bony fx; deficiency related to inadequate sun exposure, steatorrhea, severe liver or kidney disease, Crohn's disease, small bowel resection
- ▶ **Iodine** - hypothyroidism, thyroid hyperplasia and hypertrophy
- ▶ **Magnesium** - tremor, myoclonic jerks, ataxia, tetany, coma, ventricular arrhythmias, hypotension, cardiac arrest; deficiency seen in malabsorption, urinary losses
- ▶ **Sodium** - N&V, exhaustion, cramps, seizure, cardiorespiratory collapse; deficiency seen in vomiting, diarrhea, diuresis, salt-wasting renal dz, fistula, adrenal insufficiency, free water excess
- ▶ **Potassium** - confusion, lethargy, weakness, cramps, myalgias, arrhythmia, glucose intolerance, N&V, diarrhea, ileus, gastroparesis
- ▶ **Calcium** - + Chovstek's or Trousseau's sign, tetany, hyperreflexia, paresthesia, seizure, mental status changes, increased intracranial pressure, bradycardia, heart block, choreoathetotic movements
- ▶ **Phosphorus** - hemolysis, encephalopathy, sz, paresthesia, muscle weakness, rhabdomyolysis, decreased glucose utilization, reduced oxygen delivery

Toxicity Syndromes

- ▶ **Vitamin A (retinol)** - bone pain; liver dz - hepatomegaly, ascites, cirrhosis, increased size and number of stellate (Ito) cells, fibrosis; irritability, dry skin and desquamation, myalgia/arthralgia, fatigue, HA, increased intracranial pressure; requires "mega" doses: ≥ 50 IU × months–years
- ▶ **Vitamin E (tocopherol)** - uncommon; bleeding, decreased level of vit K-dependent clotting factors, impaired immune function, promotion of tumor growth, exacerbation of preexisting autoimmune dz; pharmacologic doses: protective for cardio- and cerebrovascular dz

▶ **Carotenes** - yellow-orange skin; lycopene (found in tomatoes) associated with decreased risk of gastric, colon, and prostate ca

▶ **Vitamin K** - hemolytic anemia and hypobilirubinemia in infants; impaired action of oral anticoagulants

▶ **Thiamine (B₁)** - no evidence for toxicity due to rapid excretion of excess amounts

▶ **Riboflavin (B₂)** - toxicity syndrome almost nonexistent

▶ **Niacin (nicotinic acid; B₃)** - hepatic injury, flushing, GI disturbances, burning of hands and feet

▶ **Pyridoxine (B₆)** - peripheral neuropathy with megadoses

▶ **Cobalamin (B₁₂)** - none

▶ **Folate (folic acid)** - extremely rare, if at all

▶ **Ascorbic acid (vitamin C)** - osmotic diarrhea, renal calculi, iron overload, xerostomia, infertility secondary to decreased semen

▶ **Zinc** - largely unknown; leads to copper malabsorption and deficiency

▶ **Copper** - cholestasis; increased levels seen with estrogens related to increased ceruloplasmin

▶ **Selenium** - alopecia, N&V, abnormal nails, emotional lability, peripheral neuropathy, lassitude, garlic odor to breath, dermatitis; occupational - lung and nasal carcinoma

▶ **Chromium** - occupational: renal failure, dermatitis, lung ca

▶ **Manganese** - extrapyramidal sx: accumulates in brain with dx via MRI, cholestasis

▶ **Molybdenum** - single case report: hypermethionemia, hypouricemia, hypouricosuria, low urinary excretion of sulfate

REFERENCES

1. Seres DS. Nutritional assessment: current concepts and guidelines for the busy physician. *Pract Gastroenterol* 2003;XXVII(8):30–39.
2. Feldman M, Scharschmidt BF, Sleisenger MH. *Sleisenger & Fordtran's Gastrointestinal and Liver Disease.* 6th ed. Philadelphia: WB Saunders, 1998.
3. Yamada Y, ed. *Textbook of Gastroenterology.* 3rd ed. Philadelphia: Lippincott Williams & Wilkins, 1999.
4. Goldman L, Bennett JC, editors. *Cecil Textbook of Medicine.* 21st ed. Philadelphia: WB Saunders, 2000.
5. Howard L, Ashley C. Management of complications in patients receiving home parenteral nutrition. *Gastroenterology* 2003;124:1651–1661.
6. Clinical Practice and Practice Economics Committee. American Gastroenterological Association Medical Position Statement: short bowel syndrome and intestinal transplantation. *Gastroenterology* 2003;124:1105–1110.

7. American Gastroenterological Association Clinical Practice Committee. AGA technical review on short bowel syndrome and intestinal transplantation. *Gastroenterology* 2003;124:1111–1134.
8. Klein S. A primer of nutritional support for gastroenterologists. *Gastroenterology* 2002;122:1677–1687.

CHAPTER 22

ACQUIRED IMMUNE DEFICIENCY SYNDROME (AIDS)

AIDS

Highlights

► **Helpful in Differentiating Syndromes:**
  • site of disease in GI tract
  • symptoms and demographics
  • findings on endoscopic studies

► **Major Syndromes:**
  • diarrheal syndromes
  • ulceration
  • neoplasm

► **Miscellaneous:**
  • MAC - most common finding on liver bx in HIV/AIDS
  • Pneumocystis - liver most common extrahepatic site

TABLE 22-1
DEMOGRAPHICS/SYMPTOMS-SIGNS-LABS/DIAGNOSIS/TREATMENT

GI tract site	Features	Treatment
Esophagus	• most common sx: dysphagia, odynophagia, chest pain (CP) if diagnostic testing needed, esophagogastroduodenoscopy (EGD) procedure of choice in most cases • cytologic brushing superior to biopsy in *Candida* and HSV	
• *Candida*	• endo: creamy, white plaques overlying erythematous base	• fluconazole drug of choice (unlike ketoconazole, does not require acid milieu for absorption, fewer drug interactions, broader spectrum of activity against non-*Candida* species, higher rates of cure) • recurrence universal: fluconazole 100 mg/d as prophylaxis after one relapse • amphotericin in refractory case or patient unable to swallow; complicated by nephrotoxicity and hypokalemia
• CMV	• endo: multiple ulcers, 1 – 2 cm, located in middle & distal	• ganciclovir: complicated by myelosuppression • foscarnet: requires indwelling IV catheter, complicated by renal insufficiency, hypocalcemia
• HSV	• endo: small vesicles in middle & distal esoph replaced with punched-out coalescent ulcers with potential pseudomembrane or plaque	• acyclovir

continued

TABLE 22-1
DEMOGRAPHICS/SYMPTOMS-SIGNS-LABS/DIAGNOSIS/TREATMENT (CONTINUED)

GI tract site	Features	Treatment
• IEU (idiopathic esophageal ulcer)	• endo: single or multiple ulcers, deep with rolled edges, located in mid and distal esoph • may be complicated by perforation	• prednisone 40 mg/wk × 4 wks followed by weekly tapering of 10 mg/wk
• TB & MAC	• endo: transmural ulcers with fistulas and thickened folds • TB - usually seen early in course of AIDS • MAC - usually seen relatively late	• multidrug regimen: 1. TB - isoniazid, rifampin, pyrazinamide, and ethambutol or streptomycin 2. MAC - clarithromycin, ethambutol, rifabutin
• neoplasm	• Kaposi's sarcoma, squamous cell, lymphoma	
Stomach • Kaposi sarcoma (KS)	• involves stomach more often than any other GI organ • usually clinically silent • biopsies frequently non-diagnostic	• doxorubicin • α-interferon
• non-Hodgkin lymphoma (NHL)	• gastric outlet obstruction most common presentation • involves stomach as part of diffuse process with extensive abd disease	• CHOP (cyclophosphamide, doxorubicin, vincristine, prednisone) • modified M-BACOD (methotrexate, bleomycin, doxorubicin, cyclophosphamide, vincristine, dexamethasone)
• AIDS "gastropathy"	• ↓ acid secretion in association with antiparietal cell antibodies and gastric atrophy	
Small bowel & colon	• diarrhea in 30 – 60% of AIDS patients in N. America and Europe and 90% in developing nations • 10% incidence of chronic diarrhea	

continued

TABLE 22-1
DEMOGRAPHICS/SYMPTOMS-SIGNS-LABS/DIAGNOSIS/TREATMENT (CONTINUED)

GI tract site	Features	Treatment
Small bowel & colon *(continued)*	• small bowel: abd pain, dehydration, malabsorption, weight loss, wasting • colon: small volume or bloody diarrhea, abd discomfort, tenesmus, constipation (see Figure 22-1) • homosexual & bisexual dz more likely to have diarrhea from enteric pathogens than heterosexual and intravenous drug (IVDA) disease • diarrhea seen with greater degree of immunosuppression and higher incidence of extra-intestinal opportunistic infections • cause not found in 20%	
• *Microsporidia*	• prevalence of 10 – 30% in AIDS • sx: multiple, watery BMs, abdominal discomfort with flatulence, weight loss with good appetite, afebrile, malabsorption common, CD4 usually < 50	• ? some response to albendazole
• *Cryptosporidia*	• sx: profuse, watery diarrhea, vomiting, crampy abdominal pain, flatulence, weight loss, afebrile; malabsorption, B_{12} deficiency, and lactose intolerance common, CD4 often < 100 • mainly in jejunum and ileum • positive acid-fast stain	• no effective therapy
• *Cyclospora*	• chronic, intermittent diarrhea • disease severity related to degree of immunosuppression	• TMP-SMX • may need chronic maintenance therapy due to high recurrence rate
• CMV	• most common viral infection in GI tract in AIDS • esophagus and colon most common sites	• ganciclovir • foscarnet • cidofovir

continued

TABLE 22-1
DEMOGRAPHICS/SYMPTOMS-SIGNS-LABS/DIAGNOSIS/TREATMENT (CONTINUED)

GI tract site	Features	Treatment
	• CMV colitis: persistent or intermittent diarrhea, lower abd pain, fever, weight loss, CD4 < 150 and typically < 50, tenesmus, small volume BM with regular frequency • may also see discrete ulcers, mass lesion, obstruction, perforation, gangrene, IBD-like picture	
• HSV	• distal proctitis with severe anorectal pain, tenesmus, constipation	• ganciclovir: complicated by myelosuppression • foscarnet: requires indwelling IV catheter, complicated by renal insufficiency, hypocalcemia
• MAC	• typically indicates systemic infection • small bowel > colon • small bowel: diarrhea, abdominal pain, fever, N&V, weight loss, malabsorption • microscopically may resemble Whipple's disease since PAS positive but also positive acid-fast	lifelong combination therapy: • clofazimine • ethambutol • ciprofloxacin • rifampin • rifabutin • amikacin • clarithromycin • azithromycin
• *Salmonella* • *Shigella* • *Campylobacter*	• *Shigella* seen relatively early in course of immunosuppression; *Salmonella* & *Campylobacter* seen in advanced disease • blood culture indicated if febrile	• same as in immunocompetent except, *Salmonella* - abx indicated due to high incidence of invasive disease and extraintestinal spread • maintenance tx indicated due to high recurrence rate
• "AIDS enteropathy"	• diarrhea of varying severity often accompanied by malabsorption and weight loss	symptomatic treatment

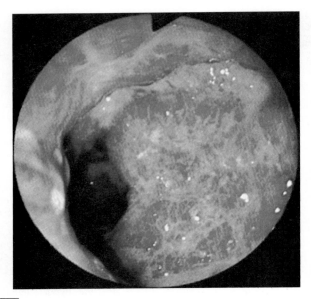

FIGURE 22-1
Kaposi sarcoma of the colon. (Reproduced with permission from Braunwald E, Fauci AS, Kasper DL, et al. *Harrison's Principles of Internal Medicine*.16th ed. McGraw-Hill, 2005.)

REFERENCES

1. Sulkowski MS, Thomas DL. Hepatitis C in the HIV-infected person. *Ann Intern Med* 2003;138:197–207.
2. Braverman IM. Skin signs of gastrointestinal disease. *Gastroenterology* 2003;124:1595–1614.
3. Brandt LJ, guest ed. Gastrointestinal disorders in AIDS. In: *Gastrointestinal Endoscopy Clinics of North America*. Philadelphia: WB Saunders, October 1998.
4. Feldman M, Scharschmidt BF, Sleisenger MH. *Sleisenger & Fordtran's Gastrointestinal and Liver Disease*. 6th ed. Philadelphia: WB Saunders, 1998.
5. Yamada Y, ed. *Textbook of Gastroenterology*. 3rd ed. Philadelphia: Lippincott Williams & Wilkins, 1999.
6. Wilcox CM. Current concepts of gastrointestinal disease associated with human immunodeficiency virus infection. *Clin Perspect Gastroenterol* 2000;3(1):9–17, .
7. Adiga GU, Dharmarajan TS, Piycumoni CS. HIV disease: gastrointestinal manifestations in older patients. *Pract Gastroenterol* 2003;XXVII(4): 24–46.
8. Sax PE. Treatment options for HIV. *Gastroenterol Endoscop News* 2002;53(1):21–25.

PART V

RELATED TOPICS

CHAPTER 23

DERMATOLOGIC MANIFESTATIONS OF GASTROINTESTINAL AND LIVER DISEASE

DERMATOLOGIC MANIFESTATIONS OF GI AND LIVER DISEASE
Highlights

GI Malignancy
▶ extramammary Paget's disease - rectal or cloacogenic ca
▶ acanthosis nigricans - gastric adenocarcinoma
▶ tylosis palmaris (autosomal dominant, hyperkeratosis of palms and soles), keratoderma - esophageal squamous cell ca
▶ Howel-Evans syndrome - esophageal ca
▶ hypertrichosis lanuginosa acquisita - gallbladder and pancreatic ca
▶ Plummer-Vinson - postcricoid esophageal ca
▶ necrolytic migratory erythema - glucagonoma
▶ flushing - carcinoid
▶ Sister Mary Joseph's nodule - gastric or colonic adenocarcinoma
▶ porphyria cutanea tarda - HCC
▶ sebaceous adenoma - colon ca
▶ Trousseau's syndrome (migratory superficial phlebitis) - pancreatic ca
▶ Virchow's node (supraclavicular lymph node) - gastric adenocarcinoma
▶ Krukenberg tumor (ovarian mets) - gastric adenocarcinoma

Nutritional Deficiency/Toxicity
▶ vit A deficiency - multiple keratotic papules on extremities
▶ vit A toxicity - alopecia, sunburn appearance, cheilosis, skin fragility, brittle nails
▶ vit B_2 (riboflavin) deficiency - seborrheic dermatitis

- vit B_3 (niacin) deficiency - pellagra
- vit B_{12} (cobalamin) deficiency - generalized hyperpigmentation of palms/soles/nails
- pernicious anemia - white hair, alopecia areata, vitiligo
- folate deficiency - lemon yellow skin
- vit C deficiency - purpura, petechiae, perifollicular hemorrhage, gingival erosions, corkscrew hairs
- zinc deficiency - acrodermatitis enteropathica, alopecia, impaired wound healing, stomatitis

Polyposis Syndromes
- Gardner's - osteomas, epidermoid cysts of scalp/face/extremities, desmoid tumors of abdominal wall
- Peutz-Jeghers - melanotic macules of lips, palms, soles, digits, periorbital skin, buccal mucosa
- Cronkhite-Canada - alopecia, onychodystrophy, hyperpigmented macules that coalesce to form plaques primarily on upper extremities
- Cowden's - facial and oral mucosal papules (tricholemmomas), oral cobblestoning, acral keratoses, lipomas, hemangiomas, neuromas, café au lait spots, scrotal appearance to tongue
- Muir-Torré - sebaceous neoplasms, basal cell ca, keratoacanthomas

GI Hemorrhage
- Osler-Weber-Rendu (hereditary hemorrhagic telangiectasia) - autosomal dominant, telangiectasias on lips, tongue, face, hands, chest, feet
- blue rubber bleb nevus syndrome - autosomal dominant, blue-colored/rubbery/compressible/nodular vascular malformations which may cause bleeding and intussusception
- Kaposi's sarcoma - GI lesions most common in small bowel and may cause bleeding and obstruction
- neurofibromatosis - autosomal dominant, café au lait spots, axillary freckles, cutaneous neurofibromas; may cause GI ulceration, bleeding, volvulus, obstruction, perforation, and intussusception

Rheumatologic Disease
- primary amyloidosis - macroglossia, pinch purpura
- scleroderma - CREST components, sclerosis of acral, perioral, and trunk areas, salt-and-pepper pigment change over sclerotic

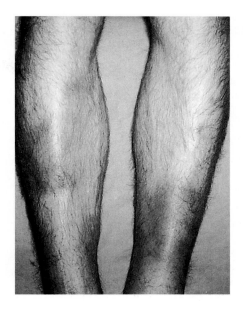

FIGURE 23-1
Erythema nodosum. (Reproduced with permission from Braunwald E, Fauci AS, Kasper DL, et al. *Harrison's Principles of Internal Medicine*. 16th ed. McGraw-Hill, 2005.)

Miscellaneous

► IBD - erythema nodosum, pyoderma gangrenosum, acquired acrodermatitis enteropathica (zinc deficiency), aphthous ulcers, angular cheilitis

► celiac sprue - dermatitis herpetiformis

► essential fatty acid (linoleic, lineic) deficiency - exfoliative dermatitis developing after long-term TPN

► cryoglobulinemia - palpable purpura

► jejunoileal bypass - pustular cutaneous vasculitis and serum sickness-like illness

REFERENCES

1. Feldman M, Scharschmidt BF, Sleisenger MH. *Sleisenger & Fordtran's Gastrointestinal and Liver Disease*. 6th ed. Philadelphia: WB Saunders, 1998.
2. Yamada Y, ed. *Textbook of Gastroenterology*. 3rd ed. Philadelphia: Lippincott Williams & Wilkins, 1999.

3. Braverman IM. Skin signs of gastrointestinal disease. *Gastroenterology* 2003;124:1595–1614.
4. Goldman L, Bennett JC, eds. *Cecil Textbook of Medicine.* 21st ed. Philadelphia: WB Saunders, 2000.
5. Bergasa NV. Itching in liver disease. *Pract Gastroenterol* 2001;XXV(8):27–37, August 2001.

CHAPTER 24

RADIOLOGIC IMAGING OF THE GASTROINTESTINAL TRACT, THE LIVER, AND BILIARY TREE

GASTROENTEROLOGY RADIOLOGY REVIEW
General Information

▶ **MRI:**
- T1: performed with GAD, fluid dark, liver bright, spleen dark
- T2: fluid bright, liver dark, spleen bright, used for MRCP
- if known primary tumor or cirrhosis, should give GAD
- useful in detection of hepatic steatosis
- T1 can distinguish HCC from non-HCC liver neoplasms (HCC and hepatic adenoma have intracellular lipid)
- can detect the presence and distribution of iron in the abdomen
- ideal for detection and characterization of hepatic cysts and hemangiomas (bright on T2 vs. mets, which are dark on T2)

▶ **Imaging of liver:**
- U/S: evaluation of size of liver and of parenchyma for diffuse infiltrative disorders, detection of mass lesions, dilation of bile ducts, and evaluation of vascular anatomy/patency/hemodynamics
- scintigraphy: evaluation of acute cholecystitis and biliary dyskinesia, confirmation of hemangioma using RBC scan and confirmation of FNH with technetium sulfur colloid
- CT: identification of liver masses, characterization of hemangiomas, staging of tumors, CT angiography to assess vascular anatomy and patency

- MRI: lesion identification/characterization/staging, pre-op evaluation for differentiation of hemangiomas from mets and detection of lesions in setting of fatty infiltration

▶ **EUS:**
  - cannot completely visualize the liver
  - superior to U/S and CT and equivalent to ERCP in diagnosis of pancreatic ca and assessment of any attendant vascular invasion
  - most accurate imaging modality for T-staging of pancreatic ca
  - better than angiography for detection of vascular involvement in pancreatic ca
  - superior to U/S, CT, MRI, ERCP for pre-op staging of ampullary ca
  - superior to U/S, CT, and MRI and equal to ERCP in detection of small (< 3 cm) bile duct tumors

Modality Specific Highlights

▶ **U/S-CT-MRI:**
  - cholelithiasis - U/S best imaging modality, "Mercedes-Benz sign" - helps detect cholesterol stones on CT
  - acute cholecystitis: U/S best imaging modality, on CT: pericholecystic fluid, perihepatitis, thickened GB wall
  - gangrenous cholecystitis - GB bright on U/S
  - emphysematous cholecystitis - CT: air in GB wall, air in GB lumen; increased risk - increased age, diabetes, ischemia
  - GB perforation - CT: nonspecific fluid, decompressed GB, stone in peritoneum; 3–15% of patients with acute cholecystitis
  - gallstone ileus - triad: pneumobilia + intestinal obstruction + stone in bowel
  - choledocholithiasis
    - U/S: biliary dilatation, sharp shadows, stones
    - CT: crescent or target sign, abrupt termination of CBD, rim calcification
    - MRCP: 95–100% sensitivity, filling defect with crescent meniscus, ductal dilation
  - recurrent pyogenic cholangitis: dilated ducts with castlike stones, pneumobilia, L lobe dominance

TABLE 24-1
IMAGING TECHNIQUES AND HEPATIC MASSES

Technique	Discussion
U/S	Noninvasive, low cost, readily available; with Doppler imaging, also provides information on vascular patency and volume and direction of flow; sensitivity to 1 cm; ideal screening technique; diagnostic for simple cysts; unable to convincingly determine etiology of solid or mixed masses; excellent technique for guided biopsy; marked obesity or bowel gas interferes with the examination; generally the screening test of first choice
CT	Radiation and contrast exposure; readily available and provides "normal anatomy" for nonradiologist; sensitivity to 1 cm; nearly isodense lesions may be missed due to volume averaging or timing of imaging to contrast injection; will screen for extrahepatic lesions simultaneously, thus identifying metastatic disease beyond the liver
Triphasic helical CT	Increased radiation exposure (must first localize lesion and then take multiple timed images); correctly identifies two-thirds of hemangiomas
CTAP	Invasive, requiring placement of angiography catheter for bolus injection; superior delineation of anatomic location of lesions to help with surgical planning; more sensitive than standard CT and will often save unnecessary surgery by identifying additional tumor nodules not noted on standard CT or US; may produce increase in false-positive findings in presence of severe cirrhosis
MRI	Totally noninvasive but very expensive; excellent biplanar images with sensitivity to 1.0 cm; more accurate than CTAP in the presence of severe cirrhosis; problems identifying lesions near the diaphragm due to cardiac motion-induced artifacts; provides additional information on vascular supply and patency
Angiography	Most invasive with high contrast dose and high radiation exposure; most expensive (along with MRI); provides most accurate information on vascular supply, patency, and flow, including pressures if needed
Nuclear medicine	Minimally invasive, less costly (except for US), and readily available; less sensitive (2.0 cm minimum); primarily useful to distinguish hepatic adenomas from focal nodular hyperplasia (due to the lack of Kupffer cells for colloid uptake in the adenomas) and identifying hemangiomas (with the Tc-99m-tagged RBC-SPECT study)[a]

[a]RBC-SPECT, Tc-99m-tagged red blood cell study utilizing single photon emission computed tomography.

- PSC: beading of bile ducts, peripheral duct pruning, globular liver, minimal duct dilation, intraductal calculi
- AIDS cholangiopathy: mural thickening, ductal irregularity, short segment strictures, papillary stenosis
- GB ca: wall thickening, polypoid mass, mass replacing GB
- cholangiocarcinoma
  - isolated ductal obstruction
  - intrahepatic: focal hepatic mass
  - hilar: lobular atrophy with biliary dilation
  - distal duct: short stricture or polypoid mass
- periampullary ca: biliary duct dilation, pancreatic duct dilation, polypoid mass
- congenital anomalies: type I choledochal cyst - fusiform dilation, fusion of CBD and PD
- pancreatic ca: focal mass, biliary and pancreatic ductal dilation, nodes; with MRCP also need MRI/MRA for staging
- mucinous cystic pancreatic ca: cannot differentiate from benign serous cystic lesion; CT: large, smoothly contoured mass; MRI: bright on T2, enhancement limited to wall
- endocrine neoplasms (islet cell): nonfunctioning tumors more commonly seen at imaging
- acute pancreatitis: enlarged, ill-defined margins, peripancreatic fluid, enhancing to non-enhancing progression implies necrosis
- chronic pancreatitis: calcification, ductal dilation
- pancreatic trauma with stricture: normal duct with sharp shift to dilated duct
- hemangioma
  - U/S: hyperechoic, well defined, no color flow within hemangioma
  - CT: low attenuation; if unenhanced, similar to aorta, central scar if large hemangioma
  - MRI: T1 - dark, T2 - isodense to CSF, post-GAD - peripheral, nodular, discontinuous enhancement
  - RBC scan: photopenic focus early with prolonged filling in on delayed scans; also seen in HCC/adenoma/FNH but have early uptake
- FNH
  - CT: early, intensely enhancing, stellate central scar; may be pedunculated

- U/S: well-demarcated mass, may be difficult to differentiate from normal liver
- RBC scan may be helpful
- MRI: isodense to liver on T1 and T2, intense enhancement with GAD
- hepatic adenoma: may see hemorrhage, early blush with GAD, US/CT/MRI - variable echogenicity/attenuation/ signal intensity
- polycystic liver/kidney: liver most common extra-renal location at 40–60%, pancreas 5–10%, autosomal dominant
- biliary cystadenoma: fluid-containing mass, ± calcification, uni/multilocular, lobulated borders, seen in middle-aged females
- liver abscess: enhancing rims
- cirrhosis: hypertrophy of L and caudate lobes and atrophy of medial and R lobes, nodular/irregular edges, enhancing lesion in cirrhotic liver implies cancer
- fatty liver:
  - U/S: diffuse hyperechoic echotexture (bright liver), increased liver echotexture compared to kidneys, vascular blurring, deep attenuation
  - CT: hepatic attenuation < blood vessels therefore *appearance* of contrast-enhanced scan in a non-contrast-enhanced CT
  - cystic fibrosis: pancreas may appear to be missing on CT due to fatty infiltration

▶ **ERCP/EUS:**
- CHD stone: ERCP preferred method of removal and requires sphincterotomy
- pancreatic head ca - "double duct" sign on ERCP
- Mirizzi's syndrome: stone in cystic duct with resultant compression of CBD
- choledochal cyst: 40% develop cancer as a result of abnormal fusion of PD and CBD, surgical resection indicated
- self-expanding wall stent: tumor growth or epithelial proliferation common cause of stent obstruction which should be treated with placement of plastic stent within stent
- primary biliary malignancy in ampulla: mass in distal bile duct
- pancreas divisum: 2–10% of population

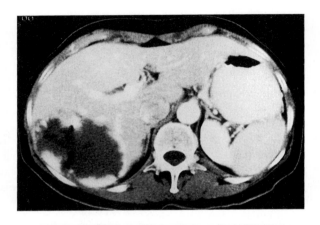

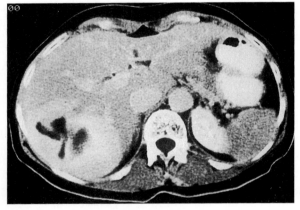

FIGURE 24-1

CT, U/S, and red cell scan with SPECT of hepatic hemangioma. (Reproduced with permission from Friedman SL, McQuaid KR, Grendell JH. *Current Diagnosis & Treatment in Gastroenterology.* Lange Medical Books/McGraw-Hill, 2003.)

- gastric stromal cell tumor (GIST): implied by calcification on EUS
- linitis plastica: overlying mucosa normal on EGD, gastric wall layers obliterated (should see 5 layers) and thickened on EUS
- islet cell tumor: homogeneous, well-defined, hypoechoic mass on EUS

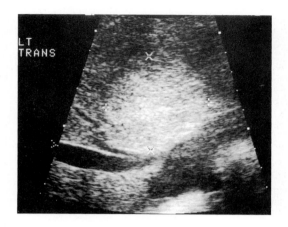

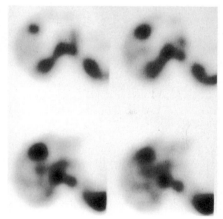

FIGURE 24-1 *continued*

- intraductal papillary mucinous tumor: ampulla dilated and patulous, extrudes mucin
- cholelithiasis: "starry sky" pattern on EUS
- ampullary ca: irregular fixed defect of distal CBD on ERCP
- PSC: "chain of beads" on ERCP
▶ **Plain Films and Barium Imaging:**
  - pneumatosis cystoides intestinalis: localized linear collections of gas on plain film; wide-based radiolucent spaces in

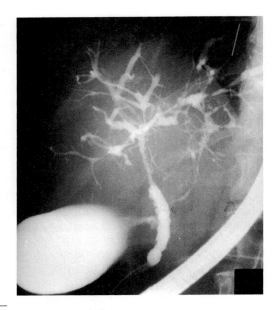

FIGURE 24-2
ERCP of PSC. (Reproduced with permission from Friedman SL, McQuaid KR, Grendell JH. *Current Diagnosis & Treatment in Gastroenterology.* Lange Medical Books/McGraw-Hill, 2003.)

    intestinal wall with smooth luminal margins on barium study
- colitis cystica profunda: radiopaque spaces in intestinal wall on barium study
- annular pancreas in infant: "double bubble sign" on plain film (air in stomach and first portion of duodenum); annular pancreas in adult - annular filling defect across 2nd portion of duodenum, symmetrical dilation of proximal duodenum, and reverse peristalsis of duodenal segment proximal to annulus on UGI
- "porcelain GB": calcified GB, high risk for GB ca, therefore cholecystectomy indicated

REFERENCES

1. Keefe EB, ed. *Atlas of Gastrointestinal Endoscopy.* Philadelphia: Appleton & Lange/Current Medicine, 1998.

2. Braunwald E, ed. *Atlas of Internal Medicine.* New York: McGraw-Hill, 2002.

3. Friedman SL, McQuaid KR, Grendell JH. *Diagnosis & Treatment in Gastroenterology.* New York: Lange Medical Books/McGraw-Hill, 2003.

4. Cope C, ed. *Current Techniques in Interventional Radiology.* 2nd ed. Philadelphia: Current Medicine, 1995.

5. Eisenberg RL. *Gastrointestinal Radiology Companion.* Philadelphia: Lippincott Williams & Wilkins, 1999.

6. Feczko PJ, Halpert RD. *Gastrointestinal Imaging Case Review.* St. Louis: Mosby, 2000.

7. Baker SR, Cho KC. *The Abdominal Plain Film with Correlative Imaging.* 2nd ed. Stamford, CT: Appleton & Lange, 1999.

8. Mishra G, Bhutani MS. EUS in pancreaticobiliary disease. *Pract Gastroenterol* 2001;XXV(3):25–42.

9. Massey NH, Nicki N. Clinical impact and safety of EUS. *Pract Gastroenterol* 2001;XXV(6):29–36.

10. Brugge W, Bounds B. Endoscopic ultrasound: its role in esophageal malignancies. *Pract Gastroenterol* 2002;XXVI(1):24–33.

11. Parasher VK. EUS of the upper GI tract: esophageal and gastric cancer staging, submucosal lesions and prominent gastric folds. *Pract Gastroenterol* 2000;XXIV(11):38–55.

12. Junquera F, Quiroga S, Saperas E, et al. Accuracy of helical computed tomographic angiography for the diagnosis of colonic angiodysplasia. *Gastroenterology* 2000;119:293–299.

13. Baillie J, Paulson EK, Vitellas KM. Biliary imaging: a review. *Gastroenterology* 2003;124:1686–1699.

14. Byrne MF, Jowell PS. Gastrointestinal imaging: endoscopic ultrasound. *Gastroenterology* 2002;122:1631–1648.

15. Saadeh S, Younossi ZM, Remer EM. The utility of radiological imaging in nonalcoholic fatty liver disease. *Gastroenterology* 2002;123:745–750.

16. Coakley FV, Qayyum A. Magnetic resonance cholangiopancreatography. *Gastrointest Endoscop* 2002;55(7):S2–S12.

17. Levine MS, Rubesin SE, Laufer I, et al. Barium studies. *Gastrointest Endoscop* 2002;55(7):S16–S24.

18. Yee J. Virtual colonoscopy (CT and MR colonography). *Gastrointest Endoscop* 2002;55(7):S25–S32.

19. Horton KM, Fishman EK. CT angiography of the GI tract. *Gastrointest Endoscop* 2002;55(7):S37–S41.

20. Anderson CM. GI magnetic resonance angiography. *Gastrointest Endoscop* 2002;55(7):S42–S48.

21. Pham KH, Ramaswamy MR, Hawkins RA. Advances in positron emission tomography imaging for the GI tract. *Gastrointest Endoscop* 2002;S53–S63.

22. Rosch T, Meining A, Fruhmorgen S, et al. A prospective comparison of the diagnostic accuracy of ERCP, MRCP, CT, and EUS in biliary strictures. *Gastrointest Endoscop* 2002;55(7):870–876.

23. Schwartz DA, Harewood GC, Wiersema MJ. EUS for rectal disease. *Gastrointest Endoscop* 2002;56(1):100–109.

24. Lightdale CA, guest ed. Advances in endoscopic ultrasound. *Gastrointest Endoscop* 2002;54(4):S2–S97.
25. Dachman AH, guest editor. Radiologic imaging in gastroenterology. In: *Gastroenterology Clinics of North America*. Philadelphia: WB Saunders, September 2002.
26. Kimmey MB, guest editor. The NIH state-of-the-science conference: ERCP for diagnosis and therapy. *Gastrointest Endoscop* 2002;56(6):S157–S302.
27. Zoler ML. MRI can rule out bile duct blockage. *Intern Med News* 2003;36(16):1–5.

CHAPTER 25

PATHOLOGY OF THE GASTROINTESTINAL TRACT, LIVER, AND BILIARY TREE

GASTROENTEROLOGY PATHOLOGY REVIEW

Highlights

▶ **Esophagus:**
- normal: prominent lamina propria, inner circle, outer longitudinal
- HSV - nuclear inclusion in squamous epithelium, ground glass, cells stuck together
- CMV - giant cell with big nucleus, affected cells in stroma
- reflux esophagitis - nonspecific, thickening, elongation, hypertrophy
- Barrett's- columnar intestinal metaplasia with goblet cells; with dysplasia - basophilic cells at surface
- high-grade dysplasia: piling up of nuclei, nuclei at surface of gland
- CMV: nuclear halo, intranuclear inclusions, intracytoplasmic inclusions (tx - acyclovir/Foscarnet if resistant)
- HSV: multinucleated giant cells, ground glass nuclei, eosinophilic Cowdry A inclusion bodies (tx - acyclovir)
- *Candida*: pseudohyphae with mucosal invasion (tx - fluconazole/amphotericin if resistant)
- XRT: epithelial hyperplasia, fibrosis
- esophagitis desiccans: shedding mucosa (causes - pill-induced, XRT, ischemia; seen in middle esoph)

▶ **Stomach:**
- normal: fundic glands, oxyntic cells, foveolar mucosa
- erosion: break in continuity of mucosa

- *Helicobacter pylori* ulcer: lymphoid nodules, positive silver stain (comma- or gull-shaped bacterium)
- follicular gastritis: *H. pylori*, gives rise to MALT *(mucosa-associated lymphoid tissue)* lymphoma
- MALT: diffuse lymphoid infiltrate without nodules, positive B cells, positive keratin stain, lympho-epithelial lesion
- chronic atrophic gastritis: drop out of glands
- dysplasia: basophilic glands at surface, no maturation at surface
- CMV: affects glandular cells
- lymphocytic gastritis: lymphoid cells in glands, no polys
- eosinophilic gastritis: eos, separation of muscle layers by eos
- Ménétrier's disease: proliferation of foveolar glands, enlarged, elongated, corkscrew, massive foveolar hyperplasia with cystic dilation
- Zollinger-Ellison syndrome (ZES): increased oxyntic mucosa, thin foveolar cells
- xanthelasma: fat-containing cells, negative PAS, looks like *Mycobacterium avium-intracellulare* (MAI) and Whipple's disease, DDx - signet ring cell ca
- GAVE (*gastric antral vascular ectasia*): ectatic vessels
- Dieulafoy's: greatly enlarged vessel
- linitis plastica: signet ring cells, gastric ca, TB, lymphoma
- carcinoid: positive chromogranin stain
- acute gastritis: poly infiltration
- chronic gastritis: lymph infiltration
- ulcer: penetration of muscularis mucosa by definition
- hypertrophic folds: Ménétrier's, lymphocytic gastritis, ZES
► **Small bowel:**
  - normal: villi:crypts = 4:1, Paneth cells imply small bowel (or R colon)
  - NSAID ulcer: clean base, few acute inflammatory cells
  - Crohn's disease: lymphoid aggregates, transmural inflammation, nonnecrotizing/noncaseating granulomas (present in only 50% of cases), thickened wall, fissuring, narrow ulcer, narrowed lumen, creeping fat, string sign on barium
  - TB: multiple caseating granulomas
  - *Yersinia*: suppurative (polys) granulomas

TABLE 25-1
INTERPRETATION OF PATHOLOGIC FINDINGS ON SMALL BOWEL BIOPSY IN MALABSORPTION

Brush border abnormalities	
Sickle-shaped organisms	Giardiasis
Basophilic dots	*Cryptosporidium*
Inclusions	Microvillous inclusion disease
Abnormal enterocytes	
Intracytoplasmic organisms	Isosporiasis
Foamy vacuolation	Abetalipoproteinemia
Lack of enteroendocrine D cells	Autoimmune polyglandular syndrome
Abnormal basement membrane collagenous band	Collagenous sprue
Villous atrophy	
Total or partial	Celiac disease, tropical sprue, bacterial overgrowth, dys-gammaglobulinemia, dermatitis herpetiformis, radiation enteritis, IPSID,[a] acute viral infections, ischemia, nongranulomatous ulcerative jejunoileitis, microsporidiosis
Lamina propria abnormalities	
Noncaseating granulomas	Crohn's disease
Infiltrating eosinophils	Eosinophilic gastroenteritis
Infiltrating malignant lymphocytes	Lymphoma, IPSID
Infiltrating mast cells	Mastocytosis
PAS-positive macrophages	Whipple's disease (bacilli on EM[b]), *Mycobacterium avium-intracellulare* (acid-fast bacilli)
Dilated lymphatics	Lymphangiectasia

[a]IPSID, immunoproliferative small intestinal disease; [b]EM, electron microscopy.

- celiac sprue: flattened villi, deep hyperplastic crypts, cuboidal epithelium infiltrated with lymphs including in crypts; "flat" mucosa (total villus atrophy) not required for diagnosis; "minimal" lesion - preserved villous architecture but with increased number of intra-epithelial lymphocytes

- MAC vs. Whipple's disease: thickened villi, villi filled with foamy macrophages, no polys, normal epithelium; Whipple + PAS stain of goblet cells and MAC: positive acid-fast stain

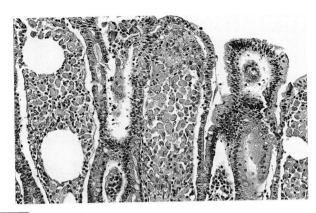

FIGURE 25-1
Histopathology of Whipple's disease. (Reproduced with permission from Braunwald
E, Fauci AS, Kasper DL, et al. *Harrison's Principles of Internal Medicine.* 15th ed.
McGraw-Hill, 2001.)

- cryptosporidiosis: basophilic brown dots on surface, no inflammation
- *Giardia*: normal villi, no inflammation, disks in spaces between
- leiomyosarcoma (GI stromal tumor - GIST): most common in stomach then small bowel, greater rate of mets in small bowel dz
- adenoma: dilated ampulla
- metastatic ca: most common ca in small bowel, especially melanoma
- carcinoid: islands of tumor in mucosa/submucosa, sclerosis, brown with immunohistochemical stain, ileum most common location in small bowel, ileum most malignant form in GI tract, appendix most common location in GI tract
- lymphoma: nodules with localization in mucosa
- lymphoid hyperplasia: common in TI

► **Colon:**
  - normal: profuse goblet cells, lymphs, plasma cells, glands down to muscularis
  - ulcerative colitis: extensive superficial ulcers, pseudopolyps, clean muscularis and submucosa, no thickening, crypt

abscesses with polys, horizontal dz (vs. vertical in Crohn's disease)

- dysplasia in IBD: increased number and size of nuclei
- lymphocytic colitis (aka microscopic colitis): lymphoid cell infiltration in glands without band of collagen
- collagenous colitis: subepithelial eosinophilic band of collagen > 10 microns on H&E, prominent lymphoid infiltrate
- diversion colitis: acute inflammatory changes in lamina propria, ↑ lymphoid follicles, superficial erosions/ulcerations, distortion of crypt architecture
- radiation colitis: connective tissue fibrosis and obliterative endarteritis with local tissue ischemia
- solitary rectal ulcer syndrome (SRUS): disorientation and thickening of muscularis, fibrosis of lamina propria, distortion of crypt architecture
- pseudomembranous colitis: mushrooming of fibrin, "volcano effect"
- angiodysplasia: dilated "varices"
- shigellosis: inflammation of lamina propria, superficial erosions, polys in epithelium, nonspecific
- amebiasis: fibrinous, necrotic, flask-shaped ulcers
- spirochetosis: fuzzy surface with black line, no inflammation, positive silver stain
- diverticulum: bleb filled with blood and feces
- pneumatosis intestinalis: large cystic areas filled with air, giant cells
- tubular adenoma: large, blue nuclei, + mucin, dysplasia
- villous adenoma: fingerlike projections
- flat adenoma: no more than 50% of the size of normal mucosa, frequently associated with high-grade dysplasia and adenocarcinoma
- adenocarcinoma: if mucinous, 50% of tumor contains mucin
- hyperplastic polyp: elongated glands, sawtooth/stellate/ branching
- Peutz-Jeghers syndrome: branching fibrinous bands with mucin-filled cells, arborizing smooth muscle with delicate appearance
- juvenile polyp: lamina propria forms infrastructure, retention cysts, no muscle seen, eroded surface, oozes blood

- Cronkhite-Canada syndrome: edematous expansion of lamina propria
- postinflammatory polyp: stalagmite/stalactite labyrinth, usually secondary to IBD
- inflammatory cloacogenic polyp: occurs in anorectal junction, part of SRUS, due to prolapse, frequently confused with cancer

► **Liver and Biliary Tree:**
- cirrhosis: collagenous scar
- amyloidosis: amorphous, eosinophilic material
- hepatitis B: ground-glass cytoplasmic changes in hepatocytes
- hepatitis C: portal tract expansion by lymphoid aggregate
- autoimmune hepatitis: rosettes, prominent component of plasma cells
- PBC: florid bile duct lesion (lymphocytic infiltration around bile duct)
- PSC: "onion-skin" fibrosis around bile duct
- Budd-Chiari syndrome: sinusoidal dilatation and RBC extravasation into hepatic cords
- ischemic liver dz: zone 3 coagulative necrosis
- alpha-1 antitrypsin deficiency: PAS-positive stain of intracytoplasmic globules
- iron overload: positive Prussian blue stain
- alcoholic liver dz: microvesicular steatosis, Mallory hyaline (eosinophilic infiltration), polys infiltration, balloon degeneration
- hepatocellular adenoma: sheets of cytologically bland hepatocytes
- focal nodular hyperplasia: centrally located scar
- angiomyolipoma: large arterial vascular structure + diffuse collection of eosinophilic cells with abundant cytoplasm + small nuclei with foci of steatosis
- peliosis hepatis: blood-filled spaces ("lakes") scattered diffusely throughout parenchyma
- HCC: trabecular pattern with trabeculae wider than normal
- acute rejection: triad - mixed chronic inflammation with eos and occasional polys + bile duct infiltration and damage + subendothelial inflammation of portal vein
- chronic rejection: ductopenia, portal tracts devoid of inflammation

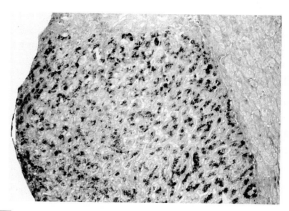

FIGURE 25-2

Liver biopsy in Wilson's disease. (Reproduced with permission from Friedman SL, McQuaid KR, Grendell JH. *Current Diagnosis & Treatment in Gastroenterology.* Lange Medical Books/McGraw-Hill, 2003.)

- CMV: intranuclear inclusion
- HSV: ground glass nuclear inclusions
- non-alcoholic steatohepatitis (NASH): macrovesicular steatosis, Mallory hyaline, zone 3 "chicken wire" fibrosis, ballooning degeneration
  - biopsy gold standard diagnostic tool
  - risk factors: obesity, diabetes
  - most have < 20 g/day of ETOH consumption
- microvesicular steatosis: Reye's syndrome, acute fatty liver of pregnancy (AFLP), valproate, TCN, aspirin, nucleoside analogs (zidovudine, didanosine, zalcitabine, fialuridine), Jamaican vomiting dz, ackee fruit, NSAIDs (naproxen, ibuprofen, ketoprofen), toxic shock syndrome, *Bacillus cereus*, ornithine transcarbamylase deficiency
- macrovesicular steatosis: NASH, ETOH, obesity, DM II, corticosteroids, estrogen, tamoxifen, amiodarone, chloroquine, Wilson's disease, jejunoileal bypass, chronic hepatitis C, Indian childhood cirrhosis
- ↑ copper: Indian childhood liver disease > Wilson's disease > PBC and PSC
- infiltrative processes → cholestasis: sarcoidosis, TB, amyloidosis, lymphoma, hepatic metastasis

234   **PART V** / RELATED TOPICS

- Mallory bodies: ETOH, ileal bypass, short bowel syndrome, obesity, diabetes, chronic cholestasis, PBC, Wilson's, Indian childhood cirrhosis, Weber-Christian disease, amiodarone

Miscellaneous

▶ **Pancreas:**
  - Johanson-Blizzard syndrome: total absence of acini
▶ **Diagnostic impact of biopsy:**
  - diagnostic (diffuse lesions): Whipple's disease, agamma-globulinemia, abetalipoproteinemia
  - may be diagnostic (patchy lesions): intestinal lymphoma, intestinal lymphangiectasia, eosinophilic enteritis, mastocy-tosis, amyloidosis, Crohn's disease, collagenous sprue, giardiasis, coccidiosis, cryptosporidiosis, MAC
  - abnormal but not diagnostic: celiac sprue, unclassified sprue, tropical sprue, viral gastroenteritis, bacterial overgrowth, radiation enteritis, folate deficiency, B_{12} deficiency
▶ **Causes of a "flat" small bowel biopsy** - celiac sprue, collagenous sprue, giardiasis, lymphoma, tropical sprue, cow's milk allergy, bacterial overgrowth, eosinophilic enteritis, viral gastroenteritis, ZES
▶ **Common mets to GI tract** - lung, stomach, breast, ovary, melanoma

REFERENCES

1. Keefe EB, ed. *Atlas of Gastrointestinal Endoscopy.* Philadelphia: Appleton & Lange/Current Medicine, 1998.
2. Braunwald E, ed. *Atlas of Internal Medicine.* New York: McGraw-Hill, 2002.
3. Friedman SL, McQuaid KR, Grendell JH. *Diagnosis & Treatment in Gastroenterology.* New York: Lange Medical Books/McGraw-Hill, 2003.
4. Bravo AA, Sheth SG, Chopra S. Liver biopsy. *N Engl J Med* 2001;344(7): 495–500.
5. Emory TS, Carpenter HA, Gostout CJ, Sobin LH. *Atlas of Gastrointestinal Endoscopy & Endoscopic Biopsies.* Washington DC: Armed Forces Institute of Pathology, 2000.

CHAPTER 26

BARIATRIC SURGERY

BARIATRIC SURGERY

► All surgical candidates should be evaluated by a comprehensive multidisciplinary team that covers medical, surgical, psychological, and nutritional issues.

► Body mass index (BMI) is used to assess obesity (calculated by dividing the weight in kilograms by the height in centimeters squared).

► Normal BMI is 18 – 24.9; BMI 25 – 29.9 is overweight; BMI 30 – 34.9 is Class 1 obese; BMI ≥ 40 (or > 35 – 39.9 with clinically significant co-morbid conditions – Class 2 obese) is morbid obesity; BMI > 50 is super density.

► Bariatric surgery is a consideration for BMI > 40 or BMI > 35 with co-morbidities.

Co-morbidities associated with morbid obesity are hypertension, type II diabetes, atherosclerosis, CHF, GB dz, hepatic steatosis, sleep apnea, osteoarthritis, venous stasis disease, GERD, and increased risk of breast, colon, and uterine ca.

Hormones of Interest

► **Grehlin** hormone is a 28-amino acid peptide secreted from the stomach, intestine, pituitary, and hypothalamus. Grehlin secretion is stimulated by fasting and low-protein diets and inhibited by leptin, interleukin-1β, growth hormone, and a high fat diet. Grehlin mediates its effect through the arcuate nucleus in the hypothalamus to increase body weight by stimulating subjective hunger (orexigenic agent) and food intake, as well as inhibiting energy expenditure and fat catabolism. Grehlin levels are inversely proportional to BMI and adiposity, change according to body weight, and rise and fall before and after meals, respectfully. In contrast to lean individuals, baseline grehlin levels are decreased in obese individuals and do not fall following a meal in obese individuals.

▶ **Leptin** hormone is produced by adipose cells. Leptin mediates its effect through the hypothalamus to decrease food intake (anorectic effect) and increase energy expenditure. Leptin inhibits neuropeptide Y, agouti-related protein, melanin-concentrating hormone and downregulates endocannabinoids and cannabinoid receptors. Leptin increases α-melanocyte-stimulating hormone, proopiomelanocortin, cocaine-regulated transcripts, and amphetamine-regulated transcripts. Most obese persons have high plasma concentrations of leptin. Though not seen in the obese person, leptin plasma concentration decreases following a meal in lean persons.

Medical Management

▶ **First-line therapy** consists of diet, exercise, and behavior modification. Low-calorie (800–1500 kcal/day) diets are recommended over very low calorie (< 800 kcal/day) diets. Sustained (30–60 minutes) exercise, at least 3× a week, can achieve at least 2% body weight loss regardless of diet. Behavior modification focuses on removing diet and exercise compliance barriers. Diet, exercise, and behavior modification in combination are more effective than diet or exercise alone. First-line therapy is usually ineffective in the morbidly obese.

▶ **Second-line therapy** consists of pharmacotherapy:
- **Sibutramine HCL monohydrate** is a serotonin reuptake inhibitor that suppresses appetite.
- **Orlistat** prevents the intestinal absorption of fat.
- Both drugs result in as much as 6% of body weight loss over 1 year. Because high weight regain occurs with drug cessation, pharmacotherapy should only be used in conjunction with lifestyle changes in a long-term weight loss program supervised by a physician.

Surgical Procedures

Restrictive Procedures

▶ **Vertical banded gastroplasty** - may be done laparoscopically or open; a 30–50 mL vertically oriented gastric pouch along with a prosthetically reinforced narrow outlet are created; complications include erosion of the prosthetic material into the gastric lumen (necessitates operative correction), creation of an outlet that is too narrow (may result in gastroesophageal reflux, solid food intolerance, and vomiting); disadvantages include less weight loss than other procedures, late failure due to pouch dilatation or poor dietary compliance; advantages include the simplicity of the procedure (no manipulation of the intestinal tract required) and the rare incidence of protein calorie malabsorption or vitamin/mineral deficiencies.

► **Laparoscopic adjustable gastric bands** - almost exclusively performed using the laparoscopic approach; the LAP-BAND device by INAMED Health is currently the only FDA-approved device for use in the United States; an inflatable and adjustable silicone band is placed around the gastric cardia to create a 15 mL pouch; the silicone band allows for adjustment of the gastric outlet diameter (reduced complications such as reflux or vomiting); complications include band slippage, gastric prolapse, decreased esophageal motility, esophageal dilatation, port complications, and band erosion; advantages include short post-op hospital stay, mortality rate < 1%

Malabsorptive Procedures
► **Biliopancreatic diversion** - performed openly; a distal gastrectomy is performed to create a 200 mL pouch, the small bowel is transected 250 cm proximal to the ileocecal valve, the distal small bowel cut end is anastomosed to the stomach and the proximal small bowel cut end is anastomosed to the ileum 50 cm proximal to the ileocecal valve; complications most often occur on a long-term basis and include fat-soluble vitamin (A, D, K, and E) deficiency, calcium deficiency (calcium, aided by vit D, is absorbed in the duodenum and proximal ileum), secondary hyperparathyroidism, bone loss, ocular abnormalities, protein calorie malnutrition, anemia, ulcers, polyarthritis, and hepatic failure; the disadvantages of this procedure include several bouts of steatorrhea per day, the dumping syndrome, and the need for long-term F/U; the advantage of this procedure is sustained weight loss over the long term.

► **Duodenal switch** - performed openly; modification of the biliopancreatic diversion procedure; the greater curvature of the stomach is resected and the pylorus is preserved (distal gastrectomy is not performed), the small bowel is transected 250 cm proximal to the ileocecal valve, the distal small bowel cut end is anastomosed to the duodenal stump, the proximal small bowel cut end is anastomosed to the ileum 50 cm proximal to the ileocecal valve; complications, F/U, and steatorrhea remain similar to biliopancreatic diversion; the dumping syndrome is not a concern and long-term weight loss is good.

Combination: Restrictive and Malabsorption Procedure

▶ **Roux-en-Y gastric bypass** - most performed bariatric procedure in North America; often performed openly but increasingly done laparoscopically; the stomach is stapled horizontally just beneath the gastroesophageal junction to create a 15 mL pouch, the small bowel is transected just distal to the ligament of Treitz, the distal small bowel cut end is used to create a gastrojejunostomy, the proximal small bowel cut end is used to form an enteroenterostomy with the Roux-limb 40 cm distal to the gastrojejunostomy; complications include GI leak, anastomotic stricture, marginal ulcers, vit B_{12} deficiency, iron-deficiency anemia; protein calorie malnutrition is rare; long-term weight loss is significantly better than gastric banding.

REFERENCES

1. 2002 Consensus Conference on Management of Obesity. *J Gastrointest Surg* 2003;7(4):433–477.
2. Levin BE, et al. Abnormalities of leptin and grehlin regulation in obesity-prone juvenile rats. *Am J Physiol Endocrinol Metab* 2003;285(5):E949–E957.
3. Hansen TK, et al. Weight loss increases circulating levels of grehlin in human obesity. *Clin Endocrinol* 2002;56(2):203–206.
4. Tschop M, et al. Circulating grehlin levels are decreased in human obesity. *Diabetes* 2001;50(4):707–709.
5. English PJ, et al. Food fails to suppress grehlin levels in obese humans. *J Clin Endocrinol Metab* 2002;87(6):2984.
6. Komer J, Aronne LJ. The emerging science of body weight regulation and its impact on obesity treatment. *J Clin Invest* 2003;111(5):565–570.
7. Fisher BL, Schauer P. Medical and surgical options in the treatment of severe obesity. *Am J Surg* 2002;184(6B):9S–16S.
8. Livingston EH. Obesity and its surgical management. *Am J Surg* 2002;184(2):103–113.
9. Norton JA, Bollinger RR, Chang AE, et al. *Surgery, Basic Science and Clinical Evidence.* New York: Springer-Verlag, 2001.

10. Schwartz SI, Shires GT, Spencer FC, et al. *Principles of Surgery*. New York: McGraw-Hill, 1999.

11. Bland KI. *The Practice of General Surgery*. Philadelphia: WB Saunders, 2002.

12. Townsend CM, Beauchamp RD, Evers BM, et al. *Sabiston Textbook of Surgery: The Biologic Basis of Modern Surgical Practice*. Philadelphia: WB Saunders, 2001.

CHAPTER 27

GASTROINTESTINAL MALIGNANCY SURVEILLANCE PROTOCOLS

GI MALIGNANCY
Surveillance Protocols

▶ Barrett's esophagus (0.5% annual risk of adenocarcinoma):
  • routine: q 2–3 years
  • low-grade dysplasia: q 6 months × 1 year then yearly if no high-grade dysplasia found
  • high-grade dysplasia: should be confirmed by 2 pathologists, esophagectomy generally recommended
▶ squamous cell esophageal ca - EGD screen in achalasia, head and neck ca, and tylosis q 1–2 years
▶ colon ca:
  • *average risk* (asxtic, age ≥ 50, no other risk factors):
    1. annual FOBT beginning at age 50; if positive, colonoscopy vs. flex + DC-BE *and*
    2. flex q 5 years; if ≤ 1 cm adenomatous polyp, patient - physician discretion; if > 1 cm adenomatous polyp, colonoscopy
    3. if African American, begin screening at age 45 and screen with a colonoscopy q 10 years (with frequency of follow-up increasing depending on findings on screening exam)
  • *moderate risk* (1st degree relative with colon ca before age 55 or adenomatous polyp before age 50):
    1. same as above but begin at age 40 (vs. American Cancer Society (ACS): colonoscopy at age 40 or 10 years earlier than youngest case with F/U q 5 years)

TABLE 27-1
COLORECTAL CANCER SURVEILLANCE FOLLOWING (PRESUMED) CURATIVE TREATMENT

Procedure	Frequency
1. H&P, FOBT, LFTs	q 3–6 mos × 2 y then q 6–12 mos × 2 y then q y
2. CEA[a]	q 2 mos × 2 y then q 4 mos × 2 y then q y
3. Sigmoidoscopy	q 6–12 mos for rectal ca
4. Colonoscopy	pre-op or during 1st y, then q 3 y × 1 then q 5 y
5. CXR[b]	q 6–12 mos × 2 y then q y

[a]CEA, carcinoembryonic antigen; [b]CXR, chest x-ray.

      2. if large/multiple adenomatous polyps - colonoscopy q 3 years

      3. if history of colon ca - post-op colonoscopy within 1 year of resection (if pre-op not performed) then at 3 years then q 5 years

- *high risk* (FAP/Gardner's syndrome, HNPCC, IBD):
  1. FAP/Gardner syndrome - flex at age 12 then annually + genetic testing
  2. HNPCC - colonoscopy q 1–2 years starting at age 20–40 then annually after age 40; consider genetic testing
  3. IBD - colonoscopy q 1–2 years after 8 years of pancolitis or 15 years of L-sided colitis

Miscellaneous: Treatment Regimens

▶ esophageal adenocarcinoma - surgical resection, ? role of pre-op 5-FU + cisplatin

▶ gastric adenocarcinoma - surgical resection; ? role of doxorubicin, mitomycin-C, or 5-FU

▶ gastric lymphoma (most common extranodal site for lymphoma, > 50% of GI lymphomas, typically non-Hodgkin's) - surgical resection with chemotherapy + XRT (4000 cGy of upper abd and 2000 cGy of liver)

▶ MALT (*mucosa-associated lymphoid tissue*) lymphoma - tx of *Helicobacter pylori*; if not curative → surgery + chemotherapy

▶ pancreatic ca - Whipple resection (pancreaticoduodenectomy); 5-FU + XRT

▶ small bowel adenocarcinoma - surgical resection

▶ small bowel lymphoma - surgical resection followed by combination chemotherapy and/or XRT

► hepatic lymphoma - lobectomy; ? followed by combination chemotherapy

► pancreatic lymphoma - surgical resection + biliary bypass procedure followed by CHOP chemotherapy

► HIV-related GI lymphoma - surgical resection + CHOP

► HCC - if localized (e.g., fibrolamellar), surgical resection; otherwise, liver transplantation if ≤ 3 lesions all of which are < 3 cm

► colon ca - surgical resection + chemotherapy if positive nodes

► rectal ca - surgical resection; surgery may be preceded by XRT and chemotherapy; + chemotherapy if penetration of bowel wall; metastatic colon ca - 5-FU + leucovorin + oritotecan

► squamous cell ca of anus - XRT + 5-FU + mitomycin

REFERENCES

1. Chung DC, Rustgi AK. The hereditary nonpolyposis colorectal cancer syndrome: genetics and clinical implications. *Ann Intern Med* 2003; 138:560–570.

2. Ransohoff DF, Sandler RS. Screening for colorectal cancer. *N Engl J Med* 2002;346(1):40–44.

3. Swaroop VS, Larson MV. Colonoscopy as a screening test for colorectal cancer in average-risk individuals. *Mayo Clin Proc* 2002;77:951–956.

4. Imperiale TF, Wagner DR, Lin CY, et al. Results of screening colonoscopy among persons 40 to 49 years of age. *N Engl J Med* 2002;346(23): 1781–1785.

5. US Preventive Services Task Force. Screening for colorectal cancer: recommendation and rationale. *Ann Intern Med* 2002;137:129–131.

6. Falk GW. Barrett's esophagus. *Gastroenterology* 2002;122:1569–1591.

7. Befeler AS, DiBisceglie AM. Hepatocellular carcinoma: diagnosis and treatment. *Gastroenterology* 2002;122:1609–1619.

8. Winawer S, Fletcher R, Rex D, et al. Colorectal cancer screening and surveillance: clinical guidelines and rationale—update based on new evidence. *Gastroenterology* 2003;124:544–560.

9. Clinical Practice and Practice Economics Committee. American Gastroenterological Association Medical Position Statement: impact of dietary fiber on colon cancer occurrence. *Gastroenterology* 2000;118: 1233–1234.

10. Spechler SJ. Barrett's esophagus. *N Engl J Med* 2002;346(11):836–842.

11. MacDonald JS, Smalley SR, Benedetti J, et al. Chemoradiotherapy after surgery compared with surgery alone for adenocarcinoma of the stomach or gastroesophageal junction. *N Engl J Med* 2001;345(10): 725–730.

12. Kapitejn E, Marijnen CAM, Nagtegaal ID, et al. Preoperative radiotherapy combined with total mesorectal excision for resectable rectal cancer. *N Engl J Med* 2001;345(9):638–646.

13. Baron TH. Expandable metal stents for the treatment of cancerous obstruction of the gastrointestinal tract. *N Engl J Med* 2001;344(22):1681–1687.

14. Adler DG, Baron TH. Endoscopic palliation of malignant dysphagia. *Mayo Clin Proc* 2001;76:731–738.

15. Morgner A, Lehn N, Andersen LP, et al. *Helicobacter heilmannii*-associated primary gastric low-grade MALT lymphoma: complete remission after curing the infection. *Gastroenterology* 2000;118:821–828.

16. Burt RW. Colon cancer screening. *Gastroenterology* 2000;119:837–853.

17. Jarvinen HJ, Aarnio M, Mustonen H, et al. Controlled 15-year trial on screening for colorectal cancer in families with hereditary nonpolyposis colorectal cancer. *Gastroenterology* 2000;118:829–834.

18. Sharms P. Short segment Barrett esophagus and specialized columnar mucosa at the gastroesophageal junction. *Mayo Clin Proc* 2001;76:331–334.

19. Bammer T, Hinder RA, Klaus A. Rationale for surgical therapy for Barrett esophagus. *Mayo Clin Proc* 2001;76:335–442.

20. Uemura N, Okamoto S, Yamamoto S, et al. *Helicobacter pylori* infection and the development of gastric cancer. *N Engl J Med* 2001;345(11):784–789.

21. Ahlquist DA, guest ed. Colorectal cancer prevention and detection. In: *Gastroenterology Clinics of North America*. Philadelphia: WB Saunders, December 2002.

22. Standards of Practice Committee. The role of endoscopy in the assessment and treatment of esophageal cancer. *Gastrointest Endoscop* 2003;57(7):817–822.

23. Tran TT, Poordad FF, Nissen N, Martin P. Hepatocellular carcinoma: an update. *Clin Perspect Gastroenterol* 2002;5(5):302–306.

24. DiBisceglie AM. Hepatocellular carcinoma. *Clin Perspect Gastroenterol* 2000;3(1):33–39.

25. Jagannath S. Hepatocellular carcinoma. *Pract Gastroenterol* 2002; XXVI(5):33–54.

26. Dural AT, El-Serag R, El-Serag HB. Hepatocellular carcinoma: epidemiology and surveillance. *Pract Gastroenterol* 2000;XXIV(10):51–58.

27. Leung WK. *Helicobacter pylori* and gastric cancer. *Pract Gastroenterol* 2001;XXV(6):38–46.

28. McGahan JP. Radiofrequency ablation of hepatocellular carcinoma. *Pract Gastroenterol* 2000;XXIV(11):21–34.

29. Parasher VK. EUS of the upper GI tract: esophageal and gastric cancer staging, submucosal lesions and prominent gastric folds. *Pract Gastroenterol* 2000;XXIV(11):38–55.

30. Sharma P, Sampliner PE. Experimental approaches to ablation of Barrett's esophagus. *Pract Gastroenterol* 2001; XXIV(11):27–35, 45–46.

31. Bernstein CN. Dysplasia surveillance in IBD. *Inflamm Dis Monitor* 2002;4(1):18–23.

32. Rex DK. Current colorectal cancer screening strategies: overview and obstacles to implementation. *Rev Gastroenterol Dis* 2002;2(supplement 1):S2–S11.

33. Yu AS, Keefe EB. Management of hepatocellular carcinoma. *Rev Gastroenterol Dis* 2003;3(1):8–24.
34. Frank BB. Updates on colorectal cancer screening and prevention. *Gastroenterol Endoscop News* 2002;53(7):61–63.
35. Alley EW, Haller DG. Advances in chemotherapy for colorectal cancer. *Gastroenterol Endoscop News* 2002;53(9):31–34.
36. Alley EW, Haller DG. Advances in chemotherapy for colorectal cancer. *Gastroenterol Endoscop News* 2001;52(7):31–34.

CHAPTER 28

MISCELLANEOUS CLINICAL PEARLS

INDICATIONS FOR ANTIBIOTIC PROPHYLAXIS FOR ENDOSCOPIC PROCEDURES

▶ Indicated in:
  1. high-risk patient + high-risk procedure
  2. moderate-risk patient + high-risk procedure
  3. PEG (percutaneous endoscopy gastrostomy) in all patients
▶ **High-risk procedures** - PEG, esoph dilation, sclerotherapy, ERCP with sphincterotomy for obstruction *low-risk procedures* - EGD ± bx, colonoscopy ± bx or polypectomy, banding
▶ **High-risk patient** - previous endocarditis episode, prosthetic cardiac valve, systemic-pulmonary surgical shunt (e.g., dialysis shunt), cyanotic congenital heart disease, synthetic vascular grafts < 1 yo
▶ **Moderate-risk patient** - rheumatic valvular dysfunction, mitral valve prolapse (MVP) with insufficiency, hypertrophic cardiomyopathy, most congenital heart lesions
▶ **Low-risk patient** - CABG (coronary artery by-pass graft), pacemaker, prosthetic joint, MVP without regurgitation

MISCELLANEOUS: ESOPHAGUS-STOMACH-SMALL BOWEL

▶ **Esophagus:**
  • pill esophagitis: mid-esoph, most common with doxycycline/quinidine/KCl; HSV - most cost common infectious esophagitis in immunocompetent
  • *Candida*: most common infectious esophagitis in immunocompromised

- caustic ingestion: most common is alkali; accidental ingestion in child < 3 yo; endo procedure of choice, if no evidence of injury in first few hours unlikely thereafter; most common products - bleach/detergent/battery/drain cleaner

► **Stomach:**
  - cardia: cardiac gland - mucus cell with secretion of mucus and pepsinogen
  - fundus and body: oxyntic gland - mucus cell (mucus), parietal cell (HCl, intrinsic factor), endocrine cell, enterochromaffin cell
  - antrum: pyloric gland - mucus cell (mucus), endocrine cell - G (gastrin) and D (somatostatin)
  - normal BAO = 15 mmol/hour in male and 10 mmol/hour in female; normal PAO_2 = 60 mmol/hour in male and 40 mmol/hour in female
  - lymphocytic gastritis: associated with celiac sprue
  - eosinophilic gastritis: infiltration of eos; sx: ulcer/early satiety/N&V/obstruction; tx: steroids
  - Ménétrier's disease: giant rugal folds, sparing of antrum, massive foveolar hyperplasia with cystic dilation; sx: abd pain, weight loss, bleeding, hypoalbuminemia
  - stress-related mucosal injury: seen in CNS injury, prolonged mechanical ventilation (> 5–7 days), coagulopathy, burns; not ICU per se
  - gastroparesis: etiology - idiopathic + diabetes most common (28%), postviral, Parkinson's disease, pseudo-obstruction; tx - erythro 125–250 mg bid, metoclopramide 40–80 mg po q day or 10 mg SC bid–qid
  - increased risk of GI event with NSAID use: 1st month of use, concomitant anticoagulant or ASA use, age > 55, ETOH, steroids
  - GIST (*gastrointestinal stromal tumor*): most common mesenchymal tumor of stomach, 10–30% malignant, 50% response rate to Gleevec (STI572), can be identified by cKIT on immunostaining
  - GAVE (*gastric antral vascular ectasia*): association seen in cirrhosis, renal failure, BMT, scleroderma; tx: ablative therapy → BCP → antrectomy + BII
  - isolated gastric varices → splenic vein thrombosis

▶ **Small bowel:**
  • resection up to 40% well tolerated, especially if duodenum, TI, and IC valve intact and normal; resection of > 50% → severe and intractable diarrhea, especially if TI and IC valve resected; resection of > 75% → severe intractable diarrhea, malabsorption, and threat to life
▶ **Duodenum:**
  • Brunner gland: bicarbonate
  • nutrient absorption:
    ■ iron: duodenum
    ■ calcium: throughout small bowel but especially duodenum
    ■ B_{12}, bile salts: ileum
    ■ fat, carbohydrate, protein, sodium, water, water-soluble vitamins except B_{12}: primarily in jejunum
    ■ folate: jejunum (with storage in the liver)
  • ileal resection: B_{12} deficiency, steatorrhea, diarrhea, stones (gallstones and calcium oxalate)
  • small bowel adenocarcinoma > carcinoid > lymphoma
  • small bowel lymphoma: ileum > jejunum > duodenum

MISCELLANEOUS
▶ **Bleeding of obscure origin:**
  • w/in reach of scope: Cameron's lesion (ulcer within hiatal hernia), esophagitis, angiodysplasia, GAVE (same as watermelon stomach)
  • beyond reach of scope: angiodysplasia
  • rate of synchronous lesions = 10%
  • push enteroscopy → 40–70% yield
  • intra-op endoscopy → 80% yield (but 50% complication rate)
  • RBC scan: need > 0.1–0.4 mL/minute for detection (500 cc over 3 days); angio: need > 0.5–1.0 mL/min (500 cc over 8 hours; 3 units PRBCs in 24 hours)
▶ **Fundoplication:**
  • Nissen: 360° wrap
  • Toupet: 270° wrap
  • Dohr: 180° wrap
▶ ETOH - 25% absorbed in stomach, 75% absorbed in duodenum

▶ "Snow White sign" on endoscopy of colon → chemical/iatrogenic colitis from colonoscopy/flex prep and/or poor rinsing of cleaning agents in scope

REFERENCES

1. Zuckerman GR, guest ed. Complications of gastrointestinal endoscopy. In: *Gastrointestinal Endoscopy Clinics of North America.* Philadelphia: WB Saunders, April 1996.
2. Feldman M, Scharschmidt BF, Sleisenger MH. *Sleisenger & Fordtran's Gastrointestinal and Liver Disease.* 6th ed. Philadelphia: WB Saunders, 1998.
3. Yamada Y, ed. *Textbook of Gastroenterology.* 3rd ed. Philadelphia: Lippincott Williams & Wilkins, 1999.
4. Clinical Practice and Practice Economics Committee. AGA Technical Review on the evaluation and management of occult and obscure gastrointestinal bleeding. *Gastroenterology* 2000;188:201–221.
5. Rebuck JA, Pisegna J. Clinical update on the prevention of stress ulcer-related gastrointestinal bleeding. *Gastroenterol Endoscop News* 2002; 53(10):57–61.
6. Jensen DM. Current diagnosis and treatment of severe obscure GI hemorrhage. *Gastrointest Endoscop* 2003;58(2):256–266.
7. Davila RE, Gaigel DO. GI stromal tumors. *Gastrointest Endoscop* 2003;58(1):80–88.
8. Clinical Practice and Practice Economics Committee. American Gastroenterological Association Medical Position Statement: short bowel syndrome and intestinal transplantation. *Gastroenterology* 2003;124:1105–1110.
9. Hawkey CJ. Nonsteroidal anti-inflammatory drug gastropathy. *Gastroenterology* 2000;119:521–535.
10. Heizer WD. Short bowel syndrome. *Clin Perspect Gastroenterol* 2002; 5(3):139–145.
11. Seidner DL. Short bowel syndrome: etiology, pathophysiology, and management. *Pract Gastroenterol* 2001;XXV(9):63–72.

QUICK GLANCE REVIEW GRIDS

CHAPTER 29

QUICK GLANCE
REVIEW GRIDS

TABLE 29-1
DRUGS COMMONLY USED IN GASTROINTESTINAL DISEASE

Drug type:	Commonly used in:	Usual dosage (po unless otherwise specified):
H2 blockers	**Acid-peptic disease**	
• Zantac (ranitidine)		150 mg bid (acute); 150 mg q d (maintenance)
• Pepcid (famotidine)		20 mg bid (acute); 20 mg q d (maintenance)
• Tagamet (cimetidine)		300 mg qid or 400 mg bid or 800 mg qhs (acute); 400 mg q d (maintenance)
• Axid (nizatidine)		150 mg bid (acute); 150 mg q day (maintenance)
Proton-pump inhibitors	**Acid-peptic disease;**	
• Prilosec (omeprazole)	**Zollinger-Ellison**	20–40 mg q d; > 60 mg q d in ZES
• Prevacid (lansoprazole)	**syndrome (ZES)**	15–30 mg q d; > 60 mg q d in ZES
• Aciphex (rabeprazole)		20 mg q d; > 60 mg q d in ZES
• Protonix (pantoprazole)		40 mg q d in erosive esophagitis
• Nexium (esomeprazole)		20–40 mg q d
Pro-kinetic/Pro-motility agents	**Acid-peptic disease;**	
• Reglan (metoclopramide)	**motility disorders; N & V**	10 mg qid 30 min ac and qhs
Antiinflammatory agents	**Inflammatory bowel disease**	
• Azulfidine (sulfasalazine)		1 g qid (acute flare); 1 g bid (maintenance)
• Pentasa (mesalamine)		1 g qid
• Dipentum (olsalazine)		1 g bid
• Asacol (mesalamine)		800 mg tid
• Rowasa (mesalamine)		500 mg suppository prn bid; 4 g suspension enema qhs
• Remicade (infliximab)		5 mg/kg IV over at least 2 h; for fistulizing Crohn's disease, 5 mg/kg IV over at least 2 h at 0 wks, 2 wks, and 6 wks

Immunosuppressive antimetabolite • Imuran (azathioprine) • 6-MP (mercaptopurine)	**IBD**	2.5 mg/kg/d 1.0–1.5 mg/kg/d
Anti-*H. pylori* agent • Helidac (bismuth 262.4 mg tablets + tetracycline 500 mg capsules + metronidazole 250 mg tablets)	*H. pylori*	Four (4) doses q day (at meals and bedtime); note: one (1) dose consists of 4 pills and each blister pack contains four (4) doses
• Tritec (ranitidine + bismuth)		
• Prevpac (lansoprazole 30 mg + amoxicillin 500 mg + clarithromycin 500 mg)		400 mg bid daily administration pack
Hepatitis agents • Intron A (interferon alfa-2b)	**Hepatitis** Hepatitis B and hepatitis C	Hepatitis B: 5 million IU q d IM or SC or 10 million IU tiw Hepatitis C: 3 million IU tiw SC or IM Body weight < 75 kg:
• Rebetron (interferon alfa-2b + ribavirin)	Hepatitis C	400 mg po q am and 600 mg po q pm + 3 million IU 3 × weekly SC Body weight > 75 kg: 600 mg po q am + 600 mg po q pm + 3 million IU 3 × weekly SC

continued

TABLE 29-1
DRUGS COMMONLY USED IN GASTROINTESTINAL DISEASE (CONTINUED)

Drug type:	Commonly used in:	Usual dosage (po unless otherwise specified):
Hepatitis agents *(continued)*	**Hepatitis**	
• peg-intron (peginterferon alfa-2b)	Hepatitis C	Body weight (kg) Dosage (µg)
		37–45 40
		46–56 50
		57–72 64
		73–88 80
		89–106 96
		107–136 120
		137–160 150
Serotonin receptor antagonist	**Irritable Bowel Syndrome**	
• Zelnorm (tegaserod maleate)		6 mg bid ac × 4–6 wks; if responsive, an additional 4–6 wk course may be a consideration

TABLE 29-2
PREGNANCY SYNDROMES

Syndrome	Trimester	Symptoms and demographics	Labs	Treatment
1. Hyperemesis gravidarum	1st (rare after 20 wks)	Severe N&V: 0.35–0.8% of pregnancies; may recur sporadically during pregnancy and in subsequent pregnancy	50% have elevated LFTs (rare for AST/ALT > 1000), mildly elevated bili < 5	IV fluids, anti-emetics (promethazine, ondansetron, droperidol)
2. Intrahepatic cholestasis of pregnancy	2nd	Severe pruritus (palms, soles; also trunk and extrem) and jaundice (1–4 wks after development of jaundice) in mother; premature delivery (60%), fetal demise; at risk for recurrence with subsequent pregnancies (60%); ? linked to MDR3 mutation; most common liver dz unique to pregnancy, more common in Chile and Scandinavia	Elevated bile acid (choly/glycine) best test, also elevated bilirubin up to 6, AST and ALT - 3–4× normal, alk phos- up to 4× normal; liver bx - bland cholestasis, bile plugs in zone 3 (central vein region), intact portal tracts	Early delivery at 36–38 wks, cholestyramine + vit K, UDCA; symptoms usually resolve a few weeks after delivery
3. HELLP *(hemolysis, elevated liver tests, & low plts)* syndrome	3rd (usually dx'd at 32–34 wks with range 22–40 wks)	Associated with preeclampsia (HTN, proteinuria, edema); asx/tic - abd pain (most common sx; usu RUQ), N&V, HA, renal failure, jaundice in 5% and seizures in severe cases, 3% mortality rate, complications - DIC, placental abruption, renal failure, ascites, pulmonary or cerebral edema, hepatic infarction - abd pain/fever/AST/ALT > 5000; potential hepatic hematoma, 0.17–0.85% or live births;	AST and ALT elevated up to 6000 and elevation prior to development of complications, plts often < 100K, low haptoglobin, elevated LDH, periph blood smear with schistocytes and burr cells;	Delivery; resolution usually w/ in days of delivery, including normal LFTs w/ in 3–5 d; plasmapheresis for pts whose plts continue to decrease after delivery

continued

TABLE 29-2
PREGNANCY SYNDROMES (CONTINUED)

Syndrome	Trimester	Symptoms and demographics	Labs	Treatment
3. HELLP syndrome (continued)		increased risk (25%) of recurrence with subsequent pregnancies; increased risk of HELLP in pts w/ gestational thrombocytopenia; 8% of uncomplicated pregnancies; 4–19% of pts with preeclampsia; 1/3 of cases occur postpartum, perinatal mortality up to 35–60%	liver bx - fibrin deposition and hemorrhage localized to periportal areas; maternal mortality up to 8% and fetal mortality up to 35%, mortality rate with rupture of hepatic hematoma > 50%	
4. Acute fatty liver of pregnancy	3rd (usually at gestational age of 35–37 wks)	Malaise, fatigue, anorexia, headache, N&V, RUQ pain, polydipsia, fulminant hepatic failure, preeclampsia present in > 50%, 10% maternal and 20% fetal mortality rate, DIC in up to 50%, pancreatitis in up to 30%, severe hypoglycemia in 25–50%, 1:13K–1:16K deliveries, linked to LCHAD deficiency - autosomal recessive so risk of recurrence in 25% of subsequent pregnancies but rare; most frequent in primigravidas (70%), avg age at onset = 27 yo, increased risk with male and twin gestations, maternal mortality rate of 15% and fetal mortality rate up to 49%	Increased LFTs but ususally < 300–1000, bili up to 40, leukocytosis, thrombocytopenia, CT and MRI - hypoattenuation of liver; liver bx - microvesicular fat deposits visualized with oil-red O	Medical and obstetric emergency - delivery, transfer to center capable of liver transplant if needed; complete recovery may take up to 1 mo, but no long-term hepatic sequelae

5. Acute viral hepatitis	All	Most common liver dz during pregnancy and most common cause of jaundice during pregnancy; higher rate of prematurity 1. HEV - case fatality rate up to 20% esp if during 3rd trimester, most cases in India, N. Africa, Mexico; GI-predominant sx, risk of transmission to fetus related to HBV DNA levels in mother 2. HAV - similar sx to nonpregnant pts, risk of prematurity in fetus 3. HBV - risk of chronicity in mother and transmission to fetus 4. HCV - transmission to fetus not yet observed 5. HSV - frequently fulminant in 3rd trimester, sx of fever, vesicular rash, and respiratory sx	HSV - marked elevations in AST and ALT without jaundice	• HBV - vaccinate infant at birth, 1 mo, and 6 mos and also give HBIG (hepatitis B immunoglobulin) (75% effective; 90% when combined with vaccine) • HSV - acyclovir
6. Chronic viral hepatitis	All	May see improvement or normalization of ALT and AST; HCV - risk of transmission to fetus at 2–4%, with risk increased with increased HCV RNA and HIV co-infection, ↓ risk of transmission if C-section delivery		

continued

TABLE 29-2
PREGNANCY SYNDROMES (CONTINUED)

Syndrome	Trimester	Symptoms and demographics	Labs	Treatment
7. Wilson's disease	All			- risk to fetus greater w/ abrupt cessation of tx - should continue tx with D-penicillamine but at lower dose, supplementation with pyridoxine; trientine safe in pregnancy
8. Cholelithiasis	All	Most common complication of pregnancy related to hepatobiliary system; cholecystectomy 2nd most frequently performed nonobstetric surgery in pregnant pt - acute cholecystitis necessary in 1 in 1000 deliveries		
9. Preeclampsia and eclampsia	Late 2nd or in 3rd trimester	Complication in 5–10% of pregnancies; HTN, edema, proteinuria, HA, hyperreflexia, visual changes, fundoscopic changes, CNS involvement with sz implies eclampsia; risk factors - preexisting HTN, 1st pregnancy, multiple gestation, extremes of child-bearing age;	Liver bx - sinusoidal fibrin deposition, periportal hemorrhage and necrosis	Mag sulfate, bed rest, anti-hypertensives, delivery in severe cases

		fetal complications - placental abruption, prematurity, intrauterine growth retardation; risk of cerebral edema, hepatic infarction and rupture, fulminant hepatic failure, acute renal failure, CHF, respiratory distress		
10. Spontaneous hepatic rupture	Late 3rd trimester and up to 48 h postpartum	Sudden onset RUQ pain, peritoneal signs, CP, shock, 50% maternal mortality rate	Decreased Hb/Hct	Intensive hemodynamic support, emergency laparotomy
11. Normal anatomy, physiology, and biochemistry during pregnancy			Decreased - albumin and protein, bili; increased alk phos, LDH, fibrinogen, transferrin, chol/TG; normal - bili, ALT slightly higher during 2nd trimester, AST, GGT, PT	

TABLE 29-3
MOTILITY SYNDROMES

Syndrome	Req'd criteria	Associated findings	Sx/signs	Treatment
1. Achalasia - occurs as result of postganglionic denervation of smooth muscle secondary achalasia (i.e., etiology known): (a) Chagas' disease - megaesoph, megaduodenum, megacolon, megaureter, cardiomyopathy ; secondary to *Trypanosoma cruzi* (b) secondary achalasia - underlying neoplasm	1. Incomplete deglutitive LES relaxation 2. Aperistalsis in smooth muscle esophagus	1. Elevated LESP 2. Elevated intra-esoph pressure	Dysphagia most prevalent sx (> 90%), regurgitation (> 70%, more common as an early sx), CP (30–50%), weight loss (60%, usually early in course), heartburn, aspiration pneumonia, regurgitant on pillow; x-ray: dilated intrathoracic esoph with air-fluid level, absence of gastric air shadow in AP view, widened mediastinum, bird's beak, sigmoid esophagus; endoscopy - scope pops through with only gentle pressure, dilated esoph; delayed on esoph emptying on radionuclide studies; increased risk of esophageal ca	1. Botox injection (30–50% response rate) 2. Pneumatic dilation (70% response rate) 3. Surgery - Heller myotomy + fundoplication prn (90% response rate)
2. Vigorous achalasia - nonperistaltic, spasm-like contractions in esophageal body	1. Incomplete deglutitive LES relaxation 2. Simultaneous deglutitive contrac-			Can try NTG, calcium channel blockers - nifedipine, diltiazem

3. Diffuse esophageal spasm (DES)	tions in smooth muscle esophagus (> 40 mm Hg) Simultaneous contractions in smooth muscle esophagus with ≥ 30% of swallows	1. Repetitive contractions (> 2 peaks) 2. Prolonged contractions (> 6 sec) 3. High amplitude contractions (> 180 mm Hg) 4. Spontaneous contractions	Corkscrew esoph on barium; CP most common sx, nonprogressive dysphagia - solids and liquids, cold > hot, weight loss related to sitophobia; regurg rare	No therapeutic agents have demonstrated efficacy for DES or any of the nonspecific disorders in controlled trials.
4. Nutcracker esophagus	1. Mean distal esophageal peristaltic amplitude > 180 mm Hg 2. Normal deglutitive LES relaxation 3. Normal peristalsis	1. Repetitive contractions (> 2 peaks) 2. Prolonged contractions (> 6 sec) 3. Increased resting LESP (> 40 mm Hg)	Noncardiac CP	Can try NTG, calcium channel blockers - nifedipine, diltiazem
5. Hypertensive LES	1. Increased resting LESP (> 40–45 mm Hg) 2. Normal deglutitive LES relaxation 3. Normal esoph body peristalsis			Can try NTG, calcium channel blockers - nifedipine, diltiazem

continued

TABLE 29-3
MOTILITY SYNDROMES (CONTINUED)

Syndrome	Req'd criteria	Associated findings	Sx/signs	Treatment
6. Nonspecific esophageal motor disorder	Peristaltic abnormalities of insufficient severity to establish any of the above diagnoses, yet not felt to be normal	1. Frequent nontransmitted contractions (> 20% of swallows) 2. Retrograde contractions 3. Repetitive contractions (> 2 peaks) 4. Low amplitude contractions (< 30 mm Hg) 5. Prolonged contractions (> 6 sec) 6. High amplitude contractions (> 180 mm Hg) 7. Spontaneous contractions 8. Incomplete LES relaxation		Can try NTG, calcium channel blockers - nifedipine, diltiazem

7. Scleroderma (CREST - calcinosis, Raynaud's syndrome, esophageal involvement, sclerodactyly, telangiectasia)	1. Incompetent LES 2. Low-amplitude contractions in smooth muscle of esoph with progression to aperistalsis	Heartburn (30–50%), dysphagia, potential stricture from reflux dz (3× more likely than in pts with routine reflux), potential odynophagia/dysphagia related to *Candida*; + ANA in 95%, anti-Scl-70 antigen in 20%, anticentromere Ab in 50%, antinucleolar antibody in 50%	Tx of reflux dz
8. Idiopathic intestinal pseudo-obstruction	1. Decreased amplitude of esoph contractions 2. Loss of peristalsis of esoph body contractions 3. Impairment of LES relaxation	Esoph complaint usually only a minor complaint	1. Bowel regimen for constipation 2. Surgical resection in select cases

TABLE 29-4
NUTRITIONAL/VITAMIN DEFICIENCY AND TOXICITY SYNDROMES

Vitamin	Sources and absorption (A)	Deficiency syndrome	Toxicity syndrome
1. Vit A (retinol)	S: pigmented vegetables and fruit, liver, enriched dairy prods A: jejunum	Poor dark (visual) adaptation, xerophthalmia, dry skin, increased infections, altered taste and smell, increased CSF pressure	Bone pain; liver disease - hepatomegaly, ascites, cirrhosis, increased size and # of stellate (Ito) cells, fibrosis; irritability, dry skin and desquamation, myalgia/arthralgia, fatigue, HA, increased intracranial pressure; requires "mega" doses - ≥ 50 IU $\times$ mos – y
2. Vit E (tocopherol)	S: vegetable oils	Hemolysis, progressive neurologic syndrome (areflexia, gait disturbance, decreased vibratory and proprioceptive sensation, gaze paresis); deficiency rare but can be seen in abetalipoproteinemia, cystic fibrosis, cirrhosis, malabsorption, biliary obstruction, excessive mineral oil ingestion	Uncommon; bleeding, decreased level of vit K-dependent clotting factors, impaired immune function, promotion of tumor growth, exacerbation of preexisting autoimmune disease; pharmacologic doses - protective for cardio- and cerebrovascular dz
3. Carotene	S: green/yellow/red vegetables		Yellow-orange skin; lycopene (found in tomatoes) associated with decreased risk of gastric, colon, and prostate cancers
4. Vit K	S: green leafy vegetables, colonic bacteria A: proximal jejunum	Prolonged PT, increased risk of hemorrhage	
5. Thiamine (B₁)	S: yeast, pork, legumes	1. Wet beriberi: unresponsive severe lactic acidosis, high-output cardiac failure, hypotension	No evidence for toxicity due to rapid excretion of excess amounts

			Toxicity
6. Riboflavin (B_2)	S: eggs, lean meat, milk, broccoli, enriched flour A: proximal small intestine, enterohepatic circulation	2. Wernicke-Korsakoff's encephalopathy: mental status changes, nystagmus, ophthalmoplegia, ataxia, coma, death Deficiency seen in alcoholics, malabsorption, severe malnutrition, prolonged fever, chronic hemodialysis	Almost nonexistent
7. Niacin (nicotinic acid; B_3)	S: meats, fish, legumes, grains, nuts A: intestine	Isolated deficiency uncommon; usually in combination with other vit deficiencies; sore throat, glossitis, cheilosis, angular stomatitis, seborrheic dermatitis, normochromic/normocytic anemia, pruritus, photophobia, visual impairment Pellagra – 4 D's: dermatitis, dementia, diarrhea, death; angular stomatitis, painful tongue; deficiency seen rarely as complication in alcoholism, malabsorption, carcinoid, Hartnup's disease	Hepatic injury, flushing, GI disturbances, burning of hands and feet
8. Pyridoxine (B_6)	S: animal protein, whole grain cereal A: jejunum; impaired by isoniazid, penicillamine, hydralazine	Isolated deficiency uncommon; usually in combination with other vit B deficiencies; peripheral neuropathy, seborrheic dermatitis, glossitis, angular stomatitis, cheilosis, seizure, sideroblastic anemia; deficiency seen in alcoholics and malabsorption	Peripheral neuropathy with megadoses
9. Cobalamin (B_{12})	S: animal sources only, produced by bacteria which are ingested by animals	Macrocytic anemia, loss of taste, glossitis, diarrhea, dyspepsia, hair loss, impotence, *neuro* – peripheral neuropathy, loss of vibratory sensation, incoordination,	None

continued

TABLE 29-4
NUTRITIONAL/VITAMIN DEFICIENCY AND TOXICITY SYNDROMES (CONTINUED)

Vitamin	Sources and absorption (A)	Deficiency syndrome	Toxicity syndrome
9. Cobalamin (B_{12}) (*continued*)	A: B_{12} complex hydrolyzed in small intestine bound to intrinsic factor and transported across ileum and stored in liver; absorbed in TI	muscle weakness and atrophy, irritability, memory loss; deficiency caused by hypochlorhydria (found in 5–15% of population >65 yo), pernicious anemia if intrinsic factor deficiency, pancreatic insufficiency, partial/gastric resection, PPIs, bacterial overgrowth, ileal disease	Extremely rare, if at all
10. Folate (folic acid)	S: ubiquitous in food; vegetables, legumes, kidney, liver, nuts A: proximal small bowel; impaired by ETOH, anticonvulsants, cholestyramine, sulfasalazine, methotrexate	Neural tube defects in fetus, megaloblastic anemia, thrombocytopenia, leukopenia, glossitis, diarrhea, fatigue; homocystinemia - may induce/aggravate occlusive vascular dz and colon ca	
11. Ascorbic acid (vit C)	S: fruits (especially citrus) and vegetables	Scurvy - petechiae, perifollicular hemorrhage, inflamed and bleeding gums, edema, impaired wound healing, lethargy; develops after 2–3 mos of dietary deficiency; deficiency also caused by alcoholism, malabsorption, Crohn's disease	Osmotic diarrhea, renal calculi, iron overload, xerostomia, infertility secondary to decreased semen
12. Zinc	S: meat, fish A: upper small bowel; impaired by dietary binders and pancreatic insufficiency	1. *Dermatologic* - symmetrical involvement of face, scalp, perianal area, hands/feet (pustular, vesicular, bullous, seborrheic, acneiform), alopecia	Largely unknown; leads to copper malabsorption and deficiency

13. Copper	A: stomach and small bowel; impaired by zinc, iron, and molybdenum	2. *Neurologic* - personality changes, lethargy, irritability 3. *Other* - growth retardation, dysgeusia, anorexia, male infertility, impaired T cell function, night blindness Deficiency seen in malabsorption, cirrhosis, alcoholism, nephrotic syndrome, sickle cell anemia, pregnancy, pica, pancreatic insufficiency, chronic diarrhea Low zinc levels with low albumin Dietary deficiency rare - deficiencies seen in parenteral nutrition; neutropenia; hypochromic - microcytic anemia, failure of elastin and collagen cross-linking resulting in vascular rupture, emphysema, and osteoporosis; neurologic disorders; impaired immune function	Cholestasis Increased levels seen with estrogens related to increased ceruloplasmin
14. Selenium	A: small bowel	1. Keshan's disease - cardiomyopathy, age 1–9 y; low soil selenium areas of China; low blood and hair levels in Keshan's district of China 2. PPN/TPN - cardiomyopathy, proximal muscle weakness and/or painful myalgias, RBC macrocytosis, pseudoalbinism Deficiency seen in malabsorption, fistulas, alcoholism, cirrhosis, AIDS, cancer	Alopecia, N&V, abnormal nails, emotional lability, peripheral neuropathy, lassitude, garlic odor to breath, dermatitis; occupational exposure: lung and nasal carcinoma

continued

TABLE 29-4
NUTRITIONAL/VITAMIN DEFICIENCY AND TOXICITY SYNDROMES (CONTINUED)

Vitamin	Sources and absorption (A)	Deficiency syndrome	Toxicity syndrome
15. Chromium	Exists in food as chromium-nicotinic acid complex known as glucose tolerance factor	Hyperglycemia, peripheral neuropathy, encephalopathy, weight loss; deficiency seen in short bowel syndrome	Occupational exposure: renal failure, dermatitis, lung ca
16. Manganese		Abnormal glucose intolerance	Extrapyramidal sx - accumulates in brain with dx via MRI, cholestasis
17. Molybdenum	S: vegetable oils	Single case report - hypermethionemia, hypouricemia, hypouricosuria, low urinary excretion of sulfate	
18. Essential fatty acids (linoleic, linolenic and arachidonic acid)		Usually caused by fat-free TPN and appears within 3–6 wks; dermatitis - dry, scaly skin progressing to exfoliative dermatitis; alopecia, coarse hair, hepatomegaly, thrombocytopenia, diarrhea, growth retardation	
19. Short-chain fatty acids (acetate, propionate, butyrate)	Stimulate colonic blood flow, colonic fluid and electrolyte absorption, butyrate preferred fuel for colonocyte		
20. Biotin	S: abundant in food	Anorexia, nausea, dermatitis, alopecia, depression, organic aciduria; deficiency seen in diets high in egg whites, PPN/TPN deficient in biotin	

21. Vit D	S: fish liver oils, eggs, liver, dairy A: small bowel	Hypocalcemia, hypophosphatemia, bone demineralization, osteomalacia in adults, rickets in children, bony fx; deficiency related to inadequate sun exposure, steatorrhea, severe liver or kidney disease, Crohn's disease, small bowel resection
22. Iodine	A: GI tract	Hypothyroidism, thyroid hyperplasia and hypertrophy
23. Magnesium		Tremor, myoclonic jerks, ataxia, tetany, coma, ventricular arrhythmias, hypotension, cardiac arrest; deficiency seen in malabsorption, urinary losses
24. Sodium		N&V, exhaustion, cramps, seizure, cardio-respiratory collapse; deficiency seen in vomiting, diarrhea, diuresis, salt-wasting renal disease, fistulas, adrenal insufficiency, free water excess
25. Potassium		Confusion, lethargy, weakness, cramps, myalgias, arrhythmia, glucose intolerance, N&V, diarrhea, ileus, gastroparesis
26. Calcium		+ Chvostek or Trousseau sign, tetany, hyperreflexia, paresthesia, seizure, mental status changes, increased intracranial pressure, bradycardia, heart block, choreoathetotic movements
27. Phosphorus		Hemolysis, encephalopathy, sz, paresthesia, muscle weakness, rhabdomyolysis, decreased glucose utilization, reduced oxygen delivery

TABLE 29-5
ENDOCRINE SYNDROMES

Syndrome	Symptoms and demographics	Features (F) and diagnosis (Dx)	Treatment
1. Insulinoma	Most common symptomatic tumor of the pancreas; sx due to hypoglycemia and frequently associated with fasting - mild personality changes, confusion, drowsiness, visual disturbance, coma; also, diaphoresis, pallor, tachycardia	F: 70–80% of the solitary tumors of the pancreas; 5–10% malignant Dx: requires documentation of hypoglycemia (glucose < 40 mg/dL) which is associated with an inappropriate increase in plasma insulin - 72-hour fast, + if serum insulin levels are stable or increase during hypoglycemia or the insulin to glucose ratio > 0.3 or corrected insulin to glucose ratio > 0.5	1. Surgery curative in 75–90% 2. Diazoxide drug of choice (150–800 mg/d) with 60% response rate - for pts awaiting surgery or those with metastatic dz
2. Gastrinoma (Zollinger-Ellison syndrome; ZES)	Sx due to gastric hypersecretory state; most common sx include hypergastrinemia associated with peptic ulcer diathesis (> 90%) - majority in duodenal bulb, diarrhea (30–40%), and esophagitis (50–60%)	F: 85% located within gastrinoma triangle (cystic duct, 3rd portion of duodenum, isthmus of pancreas), 30–40% of tumors in duodenal mucosa, 60–80% in pancreas, 50–60% malignant, 50% multiple lesions, 25% associated with MEN-I, seen in 0.1% of DU pts Dx: gastrin > 150 pg/mL, basal acid output > 15 mmol/h, secretin test > 200 pg/mL increase in gastrin	1. Surgery when possible 2. PPIs, esp omeprazole with goal of BAO < 10 mEq/h in nonoperated pts and < 5 mEq/h in operated pts or those with esophagitis
3. VIPoma (Verner-Morrison syndrome)	Sx due to excessive release of vasoactive intestinal peptide; WDHA syndrome - profuse	F: most often found in pancreas (> 90%), usually large (~ 5 cm), 50% malignant	1. Electrolytes + fluid 2. Octreotide (> 80% response rate)

continued

	(1–6 L/d) *watery diarrhea* (100%), *hypokalemia* (90–100%), *achlorhydria* (70%), also dehydration, hyperglycemia (25–50%), hypercalcemia (25%), flushing (20%); also see hypomagnesemia, hypophosphatemia	*Dx:* secretory diarrhea (> 700 mL/d) which is isotonic and persists during fasting + elevated VIP level (normal = 0–170 pg/mL); usually detectable on U/S or CT	
4. Glucagonoma	Sx due to excessive release of glucagon; triad - rash + diabetes + weight loss, migratory necrolytic erythema (70–85%) - most characteristic feature, progresses over 7–14 d, occurs most commonly in areas of friction as well as face and distal extremities; glucose intolerance or diabetes (85%), hypoaminoacidemia (80–90%), weight loss (85%), anemia (85%), diarrhea (15%), thromboembolic phenomenon (20%), glossitis (15%)	*F:* majority in body and tail of pancreas, large (> 5 cm), 50–80% malignant *Dx:* elevated plasma glucagon level ≥ 500 pg/mL (normal = 0–150 pg/mL) + appropriate clinical scenario; usually detectable on U/S or CT	1. Correction of hypoaminoacidemia 2. Octreotide (> 75% response rate)

TABLE 29-5
ENDOCRINE SYNDROMES (CONTINUED)

Syndrome	Symptoms and demographics	Features (F) and diagnosis (Dx)	Treatment
5. Somatostatinoma	Sx due to excessive release of somatostatin; if pancreatic tumor - triad of gallstones (95%), diabetes (95%), and diarrhea (92%); also steatorrhea (80%), hypochlorhydria (85%) weight loss (90%); if intestinal tumor - weight loss (70%), gallbladder dz (40%), diarrhea (38%), diabetes (20%), hypochlorhydria (17%), steatorrhea (12%); association with von Hippel-Lindau syndrome and von Recklinghausen disease	*F:* body of pancreas (56%), small bowel (44%), typically large (> 5 cm); > 70% malignant *Dx:* elevated somatostatin level + clinical scenario; usually detectable on U/S or CT	
6. GRFoma	Acromegaly - large extremities, coarsening of facial features, oily skin, malodorous perspiration, hypertrichosis, voice changes, visceral hypertrophy, glucose intolerance	*F:* 40% associated with ZES, 30% associated with MEN-I; frequently large (> 5 cm), > 60% malignant *Dx:* elevated GRF (growth hormone-releasing factor) level + clinical scenario; usually detectable on U/S or CT	

7. Carcinoid	Diarrhea (75%) + flushing (65%); also SBO, valvular heart disease, endomyocardial fibrosis, asthma, pellagra, bronchospasm in 10%	*F:* most common site is appendix and usually nonfunctional, most common location for functional tumor is TI; small bowel tumors usually not symptomatic with liver mets present; tumors in stomach/esophagus/lung commonly functional; rectal highly malignant and have early mets, however, if < 1 cm, endoscopic treatment curative *Dx:* midgut - elevated 5-HIAA (can get false positives with walnuts, bananas, avocados, Tylenol); foregut - elevated 5-hydroxytryptophan; OctreoScan	1. Metastatic dz → octreotide 2. Appendiceal → appendectomy 3. Rectal → endoscopic tx if < 1 cm; resection if > 1 cm 4. Small bowel → partial resection due to multicentric lesion in 30–50%
8. MEN-I (multiple endocrine neoplasia)	3 P's: pituitary adenoma (60%), hyperparathyroidism (95%), enteropancreatic neuroendocrine tumor (65%), most commonly gastrinoma > insulinoma; genetic defect in long arm of chromosome 11 (11q11-q13); multifocal tumors	*F:* autosomal dominant; gene abnormality on chromosome 11q; seen in 25% of gastrinoma pts, 40% of somatostatinoma pts, 33% of GRFoma pts; PPomas and nonfunctional tumors specifically associated with MEN-I gastrinoma 50%, insulinoma 40%, glucagonoma and VIPoma 5%	
9. Metastatic neuroendocrine tumors			VIPoma with best chemotherapeutic response; gastrinoma with worst chemotherapeutic response; chemotherapy - streptozotocin + 5-FU, with response rate of 40–60%

TABLE 29-6
GENETIC LIVER DISEASE

Syndrome	Demographic/genetic features (F) and diagnosis (Dx)	Symptoms	Treatment
1. Hemochromatosis	F: autosomal recessive, HLA-A haplotype, problem on chromosome 6; HFE gene - C282Y mutation (cysteine to tyrosine substitution at AA282) and/or H63D mutation (histidine to aspartate at AA63); hereditary hemochromatosis - usually homozygous for C282Y or heterozygous for C282Y and H63D; 1:200–1:500 white population, most common in northern European descent; 30% of females and 10% of males who are homozygotes do not have Fe overload Dx: elevated iron (> 175), total iron binding capacity (TIBC) (< 300), ferritin (> 200 ng/mL in female, > 300 in male) transferrin-iron saturation (TS: serum iron ÷ TIBC) > 45%; liver bx - > 4000 µg/g dry weight and hepatic iron index = 1.9 (hepatic iron index helps to distinguish between heterozygote and alcoholic with Fe overload from homozygote)	Hepatomegaly, elevated LFTs, fatigue, abd pain, bronzing of skin, arthralgias, impotence, diabetes, cirrhosis, cardiomyopathy; 200× increased risk of hepatocellular ca in cirrhotics; increased mortality secondary to HCC, diabetes, cardiomyopathy Dx and tx prior to development of cirrhosis results in normal life expectancy Liver bx - increased stainable iron in hepatocytes and bile duct cells with paucity in Kupffer cells	1. Phlebotomy - 500 mL weekly until mild anemia (Hct <75% of baseline) and ferritin < 50 ng/mL (may take up to 2 y) Phlebotomy may result in improvement in fatigue, LFT elevation, hepatomegaly, cardiac function, complications of portal hypertension but does not impact joint symptoms Vit C should be avoided, as it increases iron absorption 2. Liver transplantation - 1-y and 5-y survivals of 60% and 40%, respectively, with decreased survival due to infection and cardiac complications

2. Wilson's disease	*F:* autosomal recessive, male = female, 1 in 30,000; chromosome 13q14.3, involves up to 60 different mutations	Most present with hepatic and/or neuro sx, with presentation before age 5 or after age 40 rare, avg age for hepatic sx 10–14 yo and neuro 19–22 yo, chronic hepatitis, fibrosis, cirrhosis, fulminant hepatic failure, neuropsychiatric manifestations (depression, mood disorders, personality changes) Kayser-Fleischer rings, decreased alk phos, decreased uric acid, Coombs' negative hemolytic anemia, tremor, hypertonicity, choreoathetosis, parkinsonian-like features, splenomegaly, osteopenia, distal RTA, hypercalciuria, polyarthritis, CHF, arrhythmia, glucose intolerance, amenorrhea	1. Removal - penicillamine (1–2 g/d in 4 doses 30 minutes ac) or trientine (second line tx, less potent and fewer side effects than penicillamine); need pyridoxine supplement as penicillamine tx depletes stores
	Dx: low serum ceruloplasmin (< 20 mg/dL), slit-lamp exam, liver bx - hepatic copper > 250 µg/g dry weight (normal <35), urinary copper > 100 µg/24 h (normal <30 µg/24 h), serum copper < 80		May take weeks to months before response to tx; penicillamine may worsen neuropsych sx; neuropsych sx less responsive than liver dz; side effects - rash, nephrotic syndrome, hypersensitivity disorder
	Genetic screening appropriate: - children with liver and/or neuro dz - Fanconi's syndrome - decreased uric acid - Kayser-Fleischer rings - sibling	Liver bx - fatty infiltration, cirrhosis	Maintenance - zinc at 150 mg/d in 3 doses + low copper diet (avoid shellfish, chocolate, nuts, liver); urine excretion of 250–500 µg/d implies copper depleted state
		Liver presentations - (1) fulminant hepatic failure, (2) chronic hepatitis, (3) cirrhosis	2. Liver transplantation - curative

continued

TABLE 29-6
GENETIC LIVER DISEASE (CONTINUED)

Syndrome	Demographic/genetic features (F) and diagnosis (Dx)	Symptoms	Treatment
3. alpha-1 antitrypsin deficiency	F: most common genetic liver dz in infants and children; 1 in 1600–1 in 2800 live births; Z variant - PiZZ most common phenotype associated with liver dz and has 10–20% risk of liver dz Dx: phenotyping: most with chronic liver dz are homozygous for Z allele (PiZZ) or compound heterozygous for SZ (PiSZ); alpha-1 antitrypsin levels 10–15% of normal	Neonatal hepatitis, precocious emphysema, abd pain, hepatomegaly, variceal hemorrhage; high risk of HCC in cirrhotics 30% of cases have liver dz without lung dz Liver bx - PAS positive diastase-resistant globules	Liver transplantation - 65% long-term survival rate

TABLE 29-7
AUTOIMMUNE LIVER DISEASE

Syndrome	Demographic/genetic features (F) and diagnosis (Dx)	Symptoms	Treatment
1. Autoimmune hepatitis	*F*: female:male = 4–5:1, 10% of all cases of chronic hepatitis, bimodal age distribution - children and young adults (up to age 30) and 5th–6th decade; association with HLA-DR3, DR52, and DR4 antigens, C4a gene deletion seen in some young pts *Dx:* type I - + ANA, ASMA (anti-smooth muscle, anti-actin antibody) type II - + anti-LKM1 type III - + antisoluble liver Ag 1993 criteria: - LFT elevation > 6 months - 3–20-fold AST and ALT elevation - 1.5-fold elevation in serum gamma globulins - ANA > 1:40 - ASMA > 1:80 or anti-LKM1 > 1:80 - hepatitis due to Rx, virus, ETOH, hemochromatosis, Wilson's disease, and alpha-1 antitrypsin deficiency ruled out Type II more common in children	Predominant sx is fatigue, also anorexia, malaise, acute hepatitis (30%), acne, amenorrhea, arthralgias, autoimmune thyroid disease; majority with cirrhosis at time of dx ALT and AST in 100's with ALT > AST, elevated TP and globulins, may get false-positive HIV and HCV Degree of elevation of ANA or anti-smooth muscle Ab not predictive of dz severity or prognosis; low albumin and increased PT predict development of cirrhosis Liver bx - portal mononuclear and plasma cell infiltrate (interface hepatitis/piecemeal necrosis), sparing of bile ducts, bridging fibrosis, cirrhosis, balloon degeneration Fetal death in 15% of pregnancies and exacerbation of dz in 10–15% during pregnancy Nonresponders - HLA-DR3	Initial - (1) prednisone at 20–30 mg (2) prednisone at 10–20 mg + azathioprine at 50–100 mg Maintenance - (1) prednisone 5–15 mg or azathioprine at 2 mg/kg (2) prednisone at 5–10 mg + azathioprine at 50–150 mg Treatment should be for 1–2 y, and reduction in ALT, AST, and globulin levels may take 1–3 mos. Relapse occurs in 60% on withdrawal of tx; long-term tx may be necessary Liver transplantation - recurrence of dz in 15-40%; 92% 5-y survival

continued

TABLE 29-7
AUTOIMMUNE LIVER DISEASE (CONTINUED)

Syndrome	Demographic/genetic features (F) and diagnosis (Dx)	Symptoms	Treatment
2. Primary biliary cirrhosis (PBC)	*F:* 50 cases/million, 95% female, mean age of 40–50 yo, increased frequency of HLA-DRW8, 20% with other autoimmune disorders; slowly progressive with mean of 17 y to development of sx, 7 y avg time to death after development of sx, 50% 2-year survival once bili > 10 *Dx:* + AMA in 95%	Pruritus, jaundice - may subside spontaneously but becomes chronic and progressive with cirrhosis, xanthelasmas on eyelids, hands, and feet, osteoporosis with bone pain and fx, sicca syndrome in 50%, RTA in 50%, ? increased risk of breast ca, cirrhosis, increased risk of HCC; + anti-mitochondrial Ab (AMA - M2, M4, M8, M9 seen in PBC) diagnostic and seen in 95%, elevated alk phos, + ANA in 20%, steady rise of bili in cirrhosis, increased copper and urinary copper excretion, decreased albumin and increased PT with advanced disease, elevated chol in 300–400 range but frequently involves HDL elevation liver bx: - stage I: florid bile duct lesion with intense portal inflammation surrounding damaged duct - stage II: bile duct destruction and proliferation (biliary piecemeal) - stage III: progressive bile duct loss with bridging fibrosis	*General* 1. pruritus – UDCA, antihistamine, cholestyramine, rifampin 2. osteoporosis – calcium at 1300 mg/day + vit D at 5000 U/day 3. vitamin malabsorption – supplementation of vits D, A, E, K 4. hypercholesterolemia – Rx only if high LDL or VLDL liver transplantation - indicated if bili > 2 - 10, severe osteoporosis with vertebral fx or collapse, intractable pruritus, albumin < 3, end-stage liver disease, 90–95% two-year survival UDCA - slows progression to fibrosis and decreases LFTs but does not decrease time to trans-

Disease	Features	Labs / Dx	Treatment
3. Primary sclerosing cholangitis (PSC)	*F:* 50 cases/million, 75% male, mean age of 40–50 yo; 60–80% with HLA-B8 and/or HLA-DR3; also increased risk with HLA-DR3, DRw52a, 75% with co-existent UC but no correlation between clinical course of PSC and IBD and total colectomy does not impact PSC; 50% of cases move from asxtic to sxtic over course of 5 y; single greatest risk factor for cholangiocarcinoma (1% per y, ETOHA triples risk), increased risk of colon ca, median time from dx to end-stage liver dz of 12 y. *Dx:* multifocal strictures and irregularity involving intrahepatic and/or bile ducts	– stage IV: cirrhosis, positive copper stain. Jaundice, cirrhosis, weight loss, fatigue; elevated alk phos, normal - elevated AST, ALT, elevated chol, elevated serum and hepatic copper and ceruloplasmin; + ANA in 30%, + ANCA in 80%; liver bx - onion-skin cholangitis; ERCP - "chain of beads"	plant or increase survival - dose at 10 - 15 mg/kg/d. 1. Stenting of high-grade strictures with major ducts in pts with jaundice. 2. Liver transplantation tx of choice - indicated in prolonged jaundice, recurrent episodes of biliary sepsis, dominant stricture suggestive of cholangiocarcinoma (found in 15% at time of surgery), intractable pruritus, end-stage liver dz. 3. UDCA - improves LFTs and reduces risk of colonic dysplasia in patients with UC by 80%; does not reduce time to ESLD or transplant
4. Overlap syndromes autoimmune cholangiopathy = AMA negative primary biliary cirrhosis	*F:* sx similar to those in PBC, PSC, and autoimmune hepatitis, more common in female than male, mean age of 40–50. *Dx:* + antibody to carbonic anhydrase II	Elevated alk phos, normal bili, normal to elevated ALT and AST, + ANA, negative AMA and pANCA, + ASMA in 50%. Liver bx - bile duct damage and proliferation, periportal granuloma, normal ERCP with no stricture formation in large bile ducts	Dependent on sx-predominant syndrome, so may include UDCA, steroids, liver transplantation

TABLE 29-8
POLYPOSIS AND COLON CANCER SYNDROMES

Syndrome	Demographic/genetic features (F)	Symptoms/signs	Screening and treatment (Tx)
1. Familial adenomatous polyposis (FAP)	F: autosomal dominant; mutation of APC gene on chromosome 5q21; 1 in 8300–1:14,000 births; 2nd leading cause of death is ca of 2nd portion of duodenum (5–10%), 100% risk of colon ca • Gardner syndrome - if extraintestinal manifestations present • Crails syndrome - FAP variant with medulloblastoma of brain • Turcot syndrome - MMR mutation, oligopolyposis, malignant CNS tumors (glioblastoma, medulloblastoma, astrocytoma, ependymoma) • AFAP (attenuated FAP) - 6% of FAP pedigrees, 100% risk of colon ca but 10–15 y later than FAP, oligopolyposis, plethora of upper tract lesions (fundic gland polyps, duodenal adenomas, periampullary ca)	≥ 100 adenomas throughout colon extracolonic/extraintestinal manifestations: (a) markers - radiopaque jaw lesions, microadenomas, CHRPE (congenital *hypertrophy* of retinal pigment epithelium) lesions; ≥ 3 CHRPE lesions - 100% predictive value (b) extracolonic polyps - small bowel, stomach (including fundic gland re-tention polyps in 50–90%) (c) cutaneous lesions - lipoma, fibroma, sebaceous and *epidermoid cysts* (e) *extracolonic ca - periampullary ca,* hepatoblastoma, thyroid, duodenal, pancreas, brain, biliary tree; angiofibroma of nares in teenage males	*Screening:* (a) begin testing for APC gene at age 10–12 y (b) if gene testing not done, yearly flex starting at age 12 (c) after age 50, AGA guidelines for avg-risk pt (d) consider screening for hepatoblastoma from age 0–5 *Tx:* colectomy with ileoanal anastomosis at time of dx (if untx'd, avg age of death at 42 due to colon ca) Post-op F/U: - q 6 mos flex if rectum or pouch remains after surgery - upper endos with side-viewing scope q 6 mos - q4y - annual exam of thyroid + U/S - sulindac to help prevent polyp formation

continued

2. I1307K APC gene mutation	*F:* autosomal dominant, seen in Ashkenazi Jews, 1.4–1.9 fold increased risk of colon ca; 6% carrier frequency		
3. Peutz-Jeghers syndrome	*F:* autosomal dominant, mutation of STK11 gene on chromosome 19p, 93% develop at least one ca, with 54% of females developing breast ca	*hamartomatous polyps* (arborization of smooth muscle on path) in small bowel but also seen in colon and stomach, brown *macular melanin pigmentation* on lips/buccal mucosa/hands/feet/eyelids which fades at puberty - children - small bowel intussusception - adults - increased risk of ca of *breast, colon,* stomach, ovary (Sertoli cell tumor), lung, small bowel, uterus (adenoma malignum of cervix), esophagus, testes path of polyp - arborization of smooth muscle	*Screening:* (a) STK11 gene testing (b) screening in 1st degree relatives at least once early in 2nd decade of life w/ UGI w/ SBFT (small bowel follow through) (c) affected patients - upper and lower endo w/ bx and polypectomy and small bowel x-ray q2y (d) annual H&P + labs + baseline mammo at age 25 then yearly at age 40; + yearly pelvic and pelvic U/S beginning in adolescence + CA-125 starting at age 18 + breast and testicular self-exam *Tx:* surgery for sxtic polyps or polyps ≥ 1.5 cm
4. Solitary juvenile polyposis syndrome	Noninherited, no increased risk of ca	Presentation of 1–2 polyps in rectosigmoid at avg age of 4 y with rectal bleeding or anal prolapse of polyp	

TABLE 29-8
POLYPOSIS AND COLON CANCER SYNDROMES (CONTINUED)

Syndrome	Demographic/genetic features (F)	Symptoms/signs	Screening and treatment (Tx)
5. Juvenile polyposis coli	Autosomal dominant, 21% with DPC4 (also called SMAD4) on chromosome 18q21, mutation in PTEN gene; 20–70% risk of colon ca, increased risk of gastric, small bowel, and pancreatic ca as well as AVM and cardiovascular malformations	≥5 juvenile hamartomatous polyps, with up to 100's of polyps in colorectum but also seen in small bowel and stomach; usual presentation - anemia, rectal bleeding, failure to thrive, abd pain, hypoalbuminemia in late childhood/early adolescence; path of polyp - edematous mucosa with cystic dilation	*Screening:* (a) initial screening of 1st degree relatives with colonoscopy at age 12 (b) subsequent screening with flex + hemoccult q3–5y (c) gene testing not commercially available (d) complete upper and lower endo + small bowel imaging with bx of flat mucosa and polyps q1–3y + polypectomy prn *Tx:* colectomy (subtotal colectomy with ileoanal anastomosis) when surveillance not possible or persistent bleeding or refractory protein loss
6. Bannayan-Ruvalcaba-Riley syndrome (Bannayan-Zonana)	Possibly autosomal dominant; ? variant of juvenile polyposis, mutation in PTEN gene on chromosome 10q in 50–60%	Juvenile polyps, craniofacial appearance, developmental delay, macrocephaly, pigmented macules on shaft and glans of penis, lipid storage myopathy	Surgery required is most due to TNTC (too numerous to count) polyps

7. Gorlin's syndrome	Mutation of TCH gene on chromosome 9q	Multiple nevoid basal carcinomas, skeletal abnormalities, odontogenic keratinocytes, macrocephaly, intracranial calcification, craniofacial abnormalities	
8. Cowden's syndrome	Autosomal dominant, mutation of PTEN gene on chromosome 10q in 80%	Cardinal feature - *multiple facial trichilemmomas* (orocutaneous hamartomas) in > 90%, occurring around mouth, nose, eyes; variable hamartomatous involvement of GI tract (35%), skin, mucous membranes, thyroid, breast, adnexa; verrucous skin lesions of face and limbs, cobblestone-like papules of gingiva, buccal mucosa, and tongue; extragastrointestinal lesions - adenomas and cysts of thyroid (70%), *thyroid ca* (3%), fibrocystic dz and *fibroadenomas of breast* (52%), *breast ca* (28%), *GYN ca* in 60%	*Screening:* (a) annual H&P with special attention to neck (looking for thyroid dz) starting at age 18 or 5 years earlier than youngest age of diagnosis + breast exam at age 25 with mammo at age 30 or 5 years earlier than youngest age of diagnosis + endometrial bx at age 35 or 5 years earlier than youngest age of diagnosis + annual urinalysis
9. Basal cell nevus syndrome	Gastric hamartomatous polyps, basal cell ca		

continued

TABLE 29-8
POLYPOSIS AND COLON CANCER SYNDROMES (CONTINUED)

Syndrome	Demographic/genetic features (F)	Symptoms/signs	Screening and treatment (Tx)
10. Cronkhite-Canada syndrome	Nonfamilial, most cases seen in Japan	Multiple juvenile polyps in GI tract (except esoph), cutaneous hyperpigmentation, hair loss, nail dystrophy, protein-losing enteropathy; presenting sx - diarrhea from *protein-losing enteropathy*, weight loss, peripheral edema, fat and disaccharide malabsorption; path - mucosa between polyps with edema, congestion, and inflammation of lamina propria and focal glandular ectasia	Tx: (a) supportive therapy + enteral/parenteral nutrition (b) steroids if deterioration in condition (c) surgery for bleeding, ca, intussusception (d) colonoscopic screening for dysplasia and ca
11. Hyperplastic polyposis 12. Lynch syndrome (hereditary nonpolyposis colon ca) - Lynch I - multiple primary cancers restricted to colon and no family history of other cancers	Autosomal dominant, high risk of colon ca Autosomal dominant, accounts for 3% of colon ca cases, HNPCC gene mutation - hMSH2 on chromosome 2p16 and hMLH1 on chromosome 3p21 account for 95% of gene changes seen, 70–80% risk of colon ca and occurs at younger age (avg of 44), increased risk of extracolonic ca	100's of hyperplastic polyps Oligopolyposis, with polyps predominantly in proximal or R colon; phenotypic signs - café au lait spots, sebaceous glands tumors, keratoacanthomas extracolonic cas - *endometrial* (39%), *ovarian* (9%), transitional cell ca of ureter and renal pelvis, adenocarcinoma of stomach, small bowel, ovary, and biliary system	Biopsy to rule out FAP, surveillance for malignant transformation *Screening:* (a) + gene testing - colonoscopy starting at age 25 or 5 years earlier than youngest age of diagnosis, whichever comes first, and annually thereafter (b) if no genetic testing done, 1st degree relatives to have colonoscopy q1–2y starting at age 20–25 and annually after age 40

- Lynch II (Cancer Family Syndrome) – associated with ↑ familial occurrence of other forms of ca, esp breast, uterine, and ovarian	"Rule of 1-2-3": - 1 relative < 50 yo with colon ca - ≥ 2 generations affected - 3 affected relatives, one of whom is 1st degree relative of the other two		(c) annual screening for endometrial cancer beginning at age 25–35 with endometrial aspiration or transvaginal U/S *Tx:* subtotal colectomy with ileorectal anastomosis + postsurgical rectal surveillance q6 mos
13. Muir-Torré's syndrome	Variant of HNPCC	Oligopolyposis + skin lesions - characterized by either a sebaceous adenoma, sebaceous epithelioma or sebaceous ca + colon ca in 47%, also basal cell and squamous cell skin ca	
14. Turcot's syndrome	Can be seen as variant of HNPCC; mutation of mismatch repair gene	Adenomatous oligopolyposis + brain tumors (glioblastoma and astrocytoma)	

TABLE 29-9
VIRAL HEPATITIS

Hepatitis type	Demographics	Features and diagnosis	Screening and treatment
1. Hepatitis A	RNA virus - incubation: 15-45 days - transmission: oral-fecal (water, food, contact)	• acute - anti-HAV IgM positive; anti-HAV-IgM appears early and generally lasts 3-6 mos • anti-HAV IgG appears and persists for life after acute infection • highest attack rate in late childhood (ages 5-14) • fulminant hepatitis rare and more common in older ages or in pts with underlying liver dz	HAV vaccine: - 90% immunity - effective for preexposure prophylaxis - provides protection for 10 y Immune globulin: - effective postexposure - recommended for household and sexual contacts within 2 wks of exposure

2. Hepatitis B	DNA virus
	- incubation: 4 wks - 6 mos
	- transmission: parenteral, including sexual contact (30% transmission rate)
	
	Conversion to chronic dz decreases with age (100% in infants, 70% in childhood, 5% in healthy adults)
	
	worldwide - 350 million carriers (1 million in U.S.), 2 billion infected
	
	Accounts for 15% of chronic liver dz cases, increased risk for HCC in chronic dz
		• HBsAg positivity establishes diagnosis, appears about 6 wks after infection, and usually clears within 3 mos in transient dz.
		• Anti-HBcIgM positivity implies acute or reactivated infection.
		• Anti-HBsAg positivity generally detectable 3 mos after infection and infers recovery and immunity.
		• HBsAg implies infection.
		• HBeAg and HBV DNA imply HBV replication.
		• asymptomatic carrier:
		  - HBsAg positive with normal AST and ALT
		  - most HBeAg and HBV DNA negative
			HBV vaccine:
			- given at 0, 1, and 6 mos
			- protects for 5 y
			- preexposure prophylaxis; postexposure prophylaxis when combined with HBIG
			- double-dose recommended for dialysis pts
			- dialysis, ESLD, and immunocompromised less responsive
			• *general* – avoid ETOH and get HAV vaccine
			• *asymptomatic carrier* - no addn'l tx
			• *chronic:* interferon alfa-2b at 10 mm units tiw × 4 mos or 5 mm units daily × 4 mos, with goal of loss of HBeAg and HBV DNA:

continued

Chronic - persistence of HBsAg for ≥ 6 mos (highest risk in neonates born to HBV carrier who is HBeAg + and has high level of HBV DNA)

Pre-core mutant - HBsAg and HBV DNA positive with negative HBeAg, may be asxtic carrier or have progressive severe dz

- spontaneous clearance of HBsAg 1% per year
- appears not to have increased risk for HCC
- chronic:
  - HBsAg + HBeAg + HBV DNA positive
  - elevated AST and ALT
  - necroinflammatory disease on liver bx
  - 10% spontaneous loss of HBeAg and/or HBV DNA per year and 0.5% clearance of HBsAg per year with consequent reduction of risk of development of cirrhosis
  - 12% per year risk of development of cirrhosis
  - 6% per year risk of progression from cirrhosis to decompensated dz
  - 2.5% risk of development of HCC in cirrhotic dz
- associated extrahepatic disorders - polyarteritis nodosa (rare but 30–35% case fatality rate), renal dz: membranous glomerulonephritis - seen primarily in children, minimal change dz, IgA nephropathy, vasculitic glomerulonephritis

- 35–45% response rate
- 5–10% relapse rate in 1st year and will require re-tx
- 70–80% responders with flare characterized by elevation in AST and ALT at week 4–8 of therapy (may see ↑ to 1000); if accompanied by jaundice of deterioration in synthetic fxn, reduce dose or discontinue therapy
- side effects: flulike syndrome in 98%, depression, irritability
- reduce/discontinue therapy: severe granulocytopenia or thrombocytopenia
- positive predictors of response: high ALT, low HBV DNA levels, active necroinflammatory lesions on bx, female, negative HDV, HBV acquired after neonatal period, short duration of dz prior to tx, absence of immunosuppressive dz or therapies
- should not be used in decompensated cirrhosis but low dose (0.5–1 mm units daily) can be considered in Child's A or Child's B

TABLE 29-9
VIRAL HEPATITIS (CONTINUED)

Hepatitis type	Demographics	Features and diagnosis	Screening and treatment

2. Hepatitis B *(continued)*			• Lamivudine:
			  - 100 mg q d
			  - reduce dose if creatinine clearance <50
			  - inhibitor of HBV reverse transcription
			  - 15–50% of patients develop YMDD mutant after 1–3 y of therapy
			  - useful in helping to prevent recurrent HBV posttransplant
			  - ? duration of treatment of 1 year
			• HCC:
			  - small, unresectable tumor (<5 cm) or no more than 3 tumors with each <3 cm has 4-y survival rate with transplantation
			• Liver transplantation – high frequency of recurrent HBV infection in grafted liver
			alfa-interferon in same doses as HBV therapy (50% response rate and relapse common)

3. Hepatitis D	RNA virus - incubation: 3 wks - 5 mos - transmission: parenteral, including sexual contact - limited to patients with concurrent persistent HBV infection - may occur coincident with HBV acute infection or as	*Dx:* HBsAg plus HDV antibody positive	

4. Hepatitis C		
super-infection in chronic HBV infection; co-infection causes severe acute dz but low risk of chronic infection, super-infection usually results in chronic HDV and increases risk of severe chronic liver dz RNA virus (6 viral genotypes, with genotypes 1, 2, and 3 seen in U.S., genotype 1 more common in African Americans and less responsive to therapy) - incubation: 3–12 wks - transmission: parenteral and community; (3% transmission rate), most common cause of viral hepatitis in U.S.; 55–85% of acute cases progress to chronic dz; chronic - HCV antibody and HCV RNA positive and elevated AST and ALT - treatment response = RNA <50 IU/mL or > 2 logarithmic decline - 40% of transplant cases and 40% of CLD patients	• usually clinically silent for ≥ 20 y predictors of rapid disease progression - concomitant ETOH, HIV or HBV co-infection, older age at time of HCV acquisition, immunosuppressed state, hemochromatosis • extrahepatic disorders - cryoglobulinemia (immune complex vasculitis associated with joint, skin, and kidney involvement), glomerulonephritis • chronic: - 0.1–7% annual progression to cirrhosis - 3–7% annual progression from cirrhosis to decompensated liver dz - 1–4 % progression from cirrhosis to HCC (and usually not seen until 30 y of dz)	• *general:* - avoid ETOH and - get HAV & HBV vaccines • *chronic:* interferon monotherapy: - should be limited to those who can not be tx'd with combination therapy - indications: anti-HCV positive plus elevated ALT plus detectable HCV RNA plus evidence of chronic hepatitis on bx - 3MU tiw × 12 mos: 10–20% sustained response rate - lack of response at 3 mos implies nonresponder - positive predictors of response: shorter duration of dz, younger age, milder histologic features, lower levels of HCV RNA, genotypes 2 and 3, limited quasispecies diversity

continued

TABLE 29-9
VIRAL HEPATITIS (CONTINUED)

Hepatitis type	Demographics	Features and diagnosis	Screening and treatment
4. Hepatitis C *(continued)*		- moderate to severe necroinflammatory activity and/or fibrosis with progression to cirrhosis in 10 y - cirrhosis in HCV → 80% 10-y survival rate - cirrhosis in HCV with complications → 50% mortality rate over 5 y	- decrease response rate: increased age, increased duration of dz, increased HCV RNA levels, increased histologic stage, genotype 1b, increased iron load, presence of quasispecies • interferon + ribavirin - therapy of choice: - interferon in conventional doses + ribavirin 1000–1200 mg q d for 6–12 mos - genotype 1: response rate of 16% response rate at 6 mos and 28% at 12 mos - genotypes 2 and 3: response rate of 31% at 6 mos and 38% at 12 mos; 60–70% sustained response rate - better response rate in female, age < 40, viral load < 1 mm IU/mL - genotypes 1 and 4: less responsive to therapy - ribavirin side effects: hemolytic anemia - contraindicated in impaired renal function, chronic anemia - discontinuation of therapy necessary in 20% but if for < 2 wks has no adverse effect on response rate

- pegylated interferon alfa-2b:
  - approved as monotherapy as once-weekly injection at 1.5 µg/kg
  - efficacy similar to combination therapy
  - combination with ribavirin at > 10.6 mg/kg results in 45% response rate in genotype 1 and 90% response rate in genotypes 2 and 3
- liver transplantation:
  - invariable recurrence of HCV infection but < 50% with allograft damage and infection generally mild, clinically silent, and rarely progresses to hepatic failure
  - 5-y survival similar to that in pts with other indications for transplant

continued

| 5. Hepatitis E | RNA virus
- incubation: 2 - 9 wks
- transmission: fecal-oral (water, food, contact)
- occurs in endemic areas with poor sanitary conditions and with sporadic transmission among children; highest attack rate age 15–40 y
- 20% case fatality rate in pregnant women | • no chronic disease state
• serologic marker: anti-HEV (indicates current or past infection, anti-HEV IgM indicates current or recent infection) | |

TABLE 29-9
VIRAL HEPATITIS (CONTINUED)

Hepatitis A

	Hep A Antigen	IgM Hep A Antibody	Total Hep A Antibody
Acute			
Early	+++	+++	+++
Late	−	+	+++
Recovery	−	−	+++
Transmission	Enteric, can be from blood or body fluids (rarely)		
Incubation	15–50 days		

Hepatitis B

	Hep B s Antigen	Hep B s Antibody	Hep B c Antigen IgM	Hep B c Antigen IgG	Hep B e Antigen	Hep B e Antibody
Acute	+	−	+	−	+	+
Chronic	+	−	+	+	+	+
Chronic carrier	+	−	+	+	−	+
Transmission	Blood					

	Hep C Antibody	RIBA	Viral RNA
Incubation	Body fluids (semen, saliva, blood) Enteric 45–160 days		

Hepatitis C

	Hep C Antibody	RIBA	Viral RNA
Acute	±	±	+
Chronic	+	+	+
Transmission	Blood Sexual transmission possible		
Incubation	15–160 days		

TABLE 29-10
DIARRHEA SYNDROMES

Organism	Demographics	Features and diagnosis (Dx)	Treatment
Bacteria			
1. *Vibrio cholera*	• diarrhea due to toxin disruption of cAMP and prodn of PLT-activating factor • endemic in southern Asia, Africa, Latin America • source: seafood, fecally contaminated water • at risk: primarily children, pregnant women, hypochlorhydria, immunosuppressed • incubation: hours - 7 d • primary infection associated with immunity for at least 3 y	Epidemic cholera, vomiting, metabolic acidosis, altered sensorium, sz, electrolyte imbalance, death markers: ileus, arrhythmias, muscle cramps *Dx*: stool cx	Options: 1. TCN 250–500 mg qid × days 2. chloramphenicol 3. TMP-SMX 4. ampicillin
2. Non-cholera *Vibrio* (parahemolyticus)	Associated with undercooked seafood, eggs, potatoes, exposure to dogs	Self-limited diarrheal illness - dysentery, N&V, HA, fever *Dx*: stool cx with selective culture techniques	TCN in severe infection
3. *E. coli*	• 5 species • 3 species affect small bowel via enterotoxin: 1. enteroadherent 2. enteropathogenic (EPEC)	Small bowel: • self-limited watery diarrhea • EPEC (enteropathogenic) - watery diarrhea, vomiting, fever; usually seen in infants	Options: 1. TMP-SMX × 5 d 2. cipro 500 mg bid × 5 d Antimotility agents decrease sx

3. enterotoxigenic (ETEC)
- ETEC frequent cause of traveler's diarrhea
- transmission - contaminated food or water
- 2 species affect colon:
  1. enteroinvasive (EIEC)
  2. enterohemorrhagic (EHEC)
- EHEC = *E. coli* O157:H7
- EHEC source: unpasteurized dairy, undercooked beef, fecally contaminated water
- EHEC produces 2 Shiga-like toxins
- EHEC sx often localized to R side of colon, therefore may mimic ischemic colitis in elderly and intussusception or IBD in pediatric population
- EHEC causes 10% of cases of acute diarrhea and has < 1% overall mortality rate

- EIEC (enteroinvasive) - fever, malaise, watery diarrhea with blood or mucus, cramps; may see fecal RBC and WBC
- ETEC - traveler's diarrhea; *Dx*: stool cx with serotyping of Ag

Colon:
Enterohemorrhagic (EHEC) clinical syndromes:
1. hemorrhagic colitis
2. hemolytic uremic syndrome (hemolytic anemia, DIC, renal failure)
3. nonbloody diarrhea

EHEC - watery diarrhea and cramps followed by bloody diarrhea 12–24 h later, fever and vomiting in < 25%, sx 1–2 wks (with shedding of organism 4–8 wks)

EHEC complications: hemolytic uremic syndrome (in 2–7 % w / 10% mortality rate), TTP, most common in children or those with severe bleeding and WBC > 20K

EHEC *Dx*: stool cx on sorbitol-MacConkey agar, ELISA cytotoxin in stool colonoscopy with bx useful

EHEC: Antibiotics are not recommended as they may increase toxin production.

continued

TABLE 29-10
DIARRHEA SYNDROMES (CONTINUED)

Organism	Demographics	Features and diagnosis (Dx)	Treatment
4. *Listeria*	source: unpasteurized dairy prods, lunch meat at risk: pregnant women, infants, immunosuppressed, elderly, vets, lab workers	Diarrhea, mild fever - sepsis, cervical adenitis, endocarditis, arthritis, osteomyelitis, brain abscess, cholecystitis, peritonitis	Options: 1. ampicillin 2. TMP-SMX
5. *Staphylococcus aureus*	• 2nd most common cause of bacterial food poisoning • produces at least 7 enterotoxins • full recovery within 48 h • attack rate of 80–100% • gram-positive coccus	N&V and cramps followed by diarrhea *Dx:* clinical scenario, cx	Rehydration
6. *Bacillus cereus*	• gram-positive rod • 5th most common cause of food poisoning • produces toxin • resolution of sx within 48 h	Fried rice - vomiting, cramping Meat, vanilla sauce, salad, chicken soup, cream-filled baked goods - profuse watery diarrhea, cramping *Dx:* clinical scenario	Fluid resuscitation and antiemetics
7. *Campylobacter jejuni*	• transmission via oral-fecal route or contaminated milk, poultry, eggs, water	• sx 1–7 d after ingestion • nausea, anorexia, cramping, watery or bloody diarrhea • can mimic appendicitis • colitis frequent • Guillain-Barré syndrome frequent sequelae	Tx recommended for severe enteritis that lasts longer than 1 wk Rx: 1. erythro 2. TCN 3. cipro

continued

8. *Salmonella*	• 2200 serotypes of *Salmonella*
	• carrier state if stools positive at 1 y
		Typhi (typhoid fever):
		• fecal-oral contamination → food transmission: poultry, eggs, dairy, water; gallbladder reservoir
		• incidence: infants, elderly
		• increased risk: achlorhydria, sickle cell, chronic schistosomiasis, ETOH, cardiovascular dz
		• sx: prolonged fever, abd pain, diarrhea, GIB, rose spots, splenomegaly; possible perforation; resoln of sx after 4 wks
		Dx: stool culture
		
		Gastroenteritis/enterocolitis (non-typhoidal):
		• transmission: contaminated animal products (eggs, turkey, meat, milk)
		• presentations:
		  - asxtic carrier
		  - acute
		• enteric fever with bradycardia, rose spots, splenomegaly, leukopenia
		• bacteremia
		• high-risk: < 5 yo, homosexual men, DM, sickle cell, malaria, institutionalized
		• dysentery uncommon
		• self-limited illness
		• extraintestinal complications: osteo, mycotic aneurysm, meningitis
		Dx: stool culture
			Typhi:
			• tx not recommended as it prolongs excretion and increases relapse rate; if necessary, cipro or TMP-SMX
			
			Non-typhoidal:
			• indicated in severe sx, very young, elderly, pregnant women, immunocompromised, severe underlying illness
			• Rx: chloramphenicol, high-dose ampi or amox, TMP-SMX, cipro, ceftriaxone
			
			Carrier state:
			• quinolones

TABLE 29-10
DIARRHEA SYNDROMES (CONTINUED)

Organism	Demographics	Features and diagnosis (Dx)	Treatment
9. *Shigella*	4 species: *dysenteriae, flexneri, boydii, somnei* colitis caused by invading colonic epithelium and by producing enterotoxin most common in 1–4 yo, homosexual men, travelers, institutionalized	Toxin - small bowel watery diarrhea invasion - colon with dysentery; transmission - fecal-oral via contaminated hands *Sx:* begins in small bowel with fever, nausea, cramps, and secretory diarrhea followed by localization in colon with resultant ulcers and inflammation, bloody mucoid diarrhea and tenesmus, systemic toxicity may see toxic megacolon and obstruction mortality rate of 9%, usually in children < 9 yo and usually due to dehydration extraintestinal complications: hemolytic uremic syndrome, pneumonia, sz, encephalopathy, malnutrition, Reiter syndrome (triad of arthritis, urethritis, conjunctivitis) - most common in men 20–40 yo, seen 2–4 wks after infection, predilection for HLA-B27	Tx shortens duration of sx and decreases excretion of pathogens Options: 1. ampicillin 2. TMP-SMX 3. nalidixic acid 4. cipro × 5 days - drug of choice
10. *Yersinia*	• uncommon in U.S. • common in northern Europe • uncommon in U.S.	*Dx:* stool cx may see positive blood cx in AIDS *Sx:* • diarrheal syndrome • can mimic appendicitis or Crohn disease when presents as acute TI	Tx recommended in severe enteritis, mesenteric adenitis, erythema nodosum, and arthritis

- common in northern Europe
- source: contaminated milk or pork via fecal-oral route

- can cause acute or chronic colitis
- postinfectious complications: erythema nodosum, polyarthritis in HLA-B27, Reiter syndrome

Dx:
- stool cx with special cold-enrichment technique
- can also cx lymph nodes, blood peritoneal fluid but takes weeks
- serology with elevated antibody titers
- colonoscopy - aphthoid ulcers, round/oval elevations of mucosa

Options:
1. TCN
2. TMP-SMX
3. chloramphenicol
4. cipro

---

11. *Clostridium difficile*

- most common nosocomial infection of GI tract
- more common with po abx

Sx:
- fever, abd pain, diarrhea with gross or occult blood
- may develop toxic colitis/megacolon
- 12–24% recurrence rate
- risk factors for recurrence - old age, intercurrent abx, renal dz, prior recurrences
- 2–8% mortality rate with toxic megacolon
- *Dx:* stool cx

Options:
Diarrheal syndrome:
1. first line - metronidazole 250 mg po qid × 10 d
2. vancomycin 125 mg po qid × 10 days

Toxic megacolon:
1. metronidazole 500 mg IV q 6–8 h
2. to consider:
   - IV vanco
   - colonoscopic decompression
   - cecostomy
3. surgical resection prn

continued

TABLE 29-10
DIARRHEA SYNDROMES (CONTINUED)

Organism	Demographics	Features and diagnosis (Dx)	Treatment
11. *Clostridium difficile* (continued)			Recurrent diarrheal syndrome: 1. repeat course of same or alternative abx 2. cholestyramine or colestipol 3. *Saccharomyces boulardii* 4. *Lactobacillus* should avoid antidiarrheals
12. *Clostridium botulinum*	• produces neurotoxin that blocks acetylcholine • source: improperly canned foods, raw honey	Mild nausea, vomiting, diarrhea, abd pain, neuro sx: diplopia, ophthalmoplegia, dysarthria, dysphagia, dysphonia, descending weakness, paralysis, respiratory muscle paralysis; may take months to recover	Antitoxin, supportive care
13. *Clostridium perfringens*	• produces enterotoxin • source: improperly stored beef, fish, poultry, pasta salads, dairy products, Mexican food • recovery usually within 24 h	*Dx*: detection of toxin in stool or vomitus Watery diarrhea, cramping without vomiting; may see necrotizing enterocolitis *Dx*: demonstration of organisms in food or stool	Metronidazole in prolonged abx-associated diarrhea
14. *Aeromonas*	• source: contaminated water or shellfish • often seen in children	self-limited watery diarrhea with blood and mucus; extraintestinal manifestations - sepsis, meningitis, endophthalmitis, arthritis, cellulitis, cholecystitis	Role of therapy unclear but treat when sx severe; effective abx: cipro, chloramphenicol, TCN, TMP-SMX
15. *Plesiomonas*	• source: contaminated water or shellfish	self-limited watery diarrhea with blood and mucus; extraintestinal manifestations -	Role of therapy unclear but treat when sx severe;

continued

16. *Tuberculosis*	• often seen in children Only 50% with concomitant pulmonary involvement; transmission: ingestion of unpasteurized milk, pulmonary infection spread to GI tract	sepsis, meningitis, endophthalmitis, arthritis, cellulitis, cholecystitis Abd pain in 80–90%, abd mass, constipation *Dx:* colonoscopy with bx for histologic or microbiologic confirmation with acid-fast stain; may see strictures, deformed ileocecal valve (ICV), ulceration; may mimic Crohn disease or colon ca	effective abx: cipro, chloramphenicol, TCN, TMP-SMX
17. Tropical sprue	• results from persistent contamination of small bowel with toxigenic strains of coliform bacilli with overgrowth of *Klebsiella, E. coli, Enterobacter cloacae* in most • usually seen in residents or long-term visitors (> 1 y) in Africa, Middle East, Cuba, Central America, Puerto Rico, Haiti, Dominican Republic • distinguished from classic small bowel overgrowth by presence of only 1–2 species	Acute watery diarrhea with cramping and gas which becomes chronic; lactose and ETOH intolerance, folate deficiency within 2–4 mos → anorexia, weight loss and folate and B_{12} deficiency within 6 mos → megaloblastic anemia with weakness and glossitis; may also see ↓ carotene, vit A, vit D, albumin, cholesterol, calcium *Dx:* 1. ↓ D-xylose absorption 2. steatorrhea in 50–90% 3. abnormal glucose tolerance test in 50% 4. thickened and coarsened mucosal folds on small bowel barium study 5. bx: broadening and shortening of villi, infiltration of lamina propria with chronic inflammatory cells	Folate 5 mg/d + B_{12} 1000 μg/wk + TCN 250 mg qid × 6 mos

TABLE 29-10
DIARRHEA SYNDROMES (CONTINUED)

Organism	Demographics	Features and diagnosis (Dx)	Treatment
18. *Tropheryma whippelii* (Whipple's disease)	most cases - 50 yo white males 25% HLA-B27	Weight loss up to >100 lbs, diarrhea, arthralgias (migratory, large joints, precedes dx by 9 y, attacks lasting hours to days, sacroiliitis in 20–30%), fever, abd pain, occult GIB, pericarditis and endocarditis in 50–75%, systolic murmur in 25%, peripheral lymphadenopathy in 50%, oculomasticatory myorhythmia unique to Whipple disease, CNS - dementia, personality change, Wernicke syndrome, ataxia, anemia - chronic dz, folate and B_{12} deficiency, ↓ albumin, ↑ PT, abnormal D-xylose in 80% weight loss, diarrhea, fever precede dx 1–4 years *Dx:* PAS-positive bacilli in macrophages on small bowel bx (need 4–6 bx; take bx for electron microscopic eval as well)	1. TMP-SMX bid × 1 y; if sulfa allergic PCN 2. supplemental folate, Fe, B_{12}, fat-soluble vitamins 3. periodic re-eval due to not infrequent relapse esp in CNS (check CSF) 4. if CNS relapse, repeat 1-y course of TMP-SMX; if unresponsive, chloramphenicol; if non-CNS relapse, TMP-SMX × 1 y; if unresponsive, PCN
Viruses 1. Rotavirus	• RNA virus • incidence greatest in children 6–24 mos old • fecal-oral, person-to-person transmission • 80–100% of children have Ab by age 2 • 48–72 h incubation	Severe diarrhea, vomiting, profound dehydration, metabolic acidosis, electrolyte disturbance, low-grade fever, pharyngitis, otitis media *Dx:* stool antibody assay	Hydration and electrolyte replacement

continued

2. Norwalk agent	• fecal-oral, person-to-person and airborne transmission • source: contaminated water and shellfish • 24–48 hour incubation	Diarrhea with N&V, low-grade fever, cramping, myalgias, anorexia, HA No commercially available diagnostic tests	Hydration and electrolyte replacement
3. CMV	seen in immunocompromised	Self-limited colitis; dx on biopsy	Therapy not indicated in self-limited dz
4. HSV	sexually transmitted	Distal proctitis following anal intercourse; severe anal pain and discharge, urinary retention, pain in abd/buttocks/thighs *Dx:* viral isolation from culture of rectal swab or bx; flex sig helpful focal ulcers and vesicles	Acyclovir
Parasites 1. *Giardia lamblia*	• most common water-borne cause of diarrhea • transmission by direct person-to-person route with ingestion of contaminated food or water • high-risk: male homosexual, camper/hiker, day care, s/p gastrectomy, cystic fibrosis, immunosuppressive Rx, AIDS	Chronic infection in immunoglobulin deficiency *Sx:* crampy abd pain, nausea, bloating, flatulence, anorexia, explosive watery, foul-smelling, greasy diarrhea *Dx:* • cysts in stool (3 stools over 6 d due to intermittent excretion) • duodenal aspiration for trophozoites • *Giardia* antigen	Options: 1. quinacrine 100 mg tid × 7 d 2. metronidazole 250 mg tid × 7 d 3. combination of both

TABLE 29-10
DIARRHEA SYNDROMES (CONTINUED)

Organism	Demographics	Features and diagnosis (Dx)	Treatment
2. *Cryptosporidia*	• source: fecally contaminated water • outbreaks reported in day care centers, livestock/veterinary workers • can be chronic in AIDS patients	Profuse, watery diarrhea *Dx:* acid-fast or immunofluorescent monoclonal antibody stain of stool	No effective therapy
3. *Microsporidia*	Recognized as pathogen in HIV		Albendazole 400 mg bid – tid up to 3 mos
4. *Isospora belli*			1. TMP-SMX qid × 7 d then bid × 3 wks 2. sulfadiazine 4 g and pyrimethamine 35–75 mg qid + leucovorin calcium 15–25 mg q day × 3–7 wks TMP-SMX shortens duration of sx
5. *Cyclospora cayetanensis*	Source: contaminated water and raspberries, mesclun lettuce	Prolonged, watery diarrhea (4–6 wks) usually without fever, prodrome of flulike illness and profound fatigue and GERD may overshadow diarrheal illness *Dx:* positive acid-fast or safranin stain	
6. *Entamoeba histolytica*	Source: contaminated food or water	Range of sx: asxtic carrier state - severe dysentery, hepatic abscess, colicky abd pain, diarrhea alternating with constipation, may get toxic megacolon, may mimic colon ca with strictures/amebomas on DC-BE	Metronidazole 750 mg tid × 10 d with or followed by iodoquinol 650 mg tid × 20 d

		Dx: check stool or swab for cysts/trophozoites	
7. *Entamoeba coli*	Nonpathogenic strains common in homosexual men		Nonpathogenic
8. *Entamoeba hartmanni*	Nonpathogenic strains common in homosexual men		Nonpathogenic
9. *Endolimax nana*	Nonpathogenic strains common in homosexual men		Nonpathogenic
10. *Iodamoeba buetschlii*	Nonpathogenic strains common in homosexual men		Nonpathogenic
11. *Blastocystis hominis*	? Nonpathogenic ? sx correlate with # of organisms (> 5 organisms/high power field)		Metronidazole, also responds to TMP-SMX
12. *Balantidium coli*	Rare cases of chronic colitis have been described		TCN
Fungi			
1. *Candida*	Seen in immunocompromised	Colonic ulcers have been described *Dx:* biopsy	
2. Histoplasmosis	Can occur in immunocompetent	Can involve small and large bowel	
3. Paracoccidioidomycosis (S. American blastomycosis)	Seen in immunocompromised	Granulomatous inflammation resembling Crohn's disease *Dx:* biopsy	

TABLE 29-11
INTESTINAL ISCHEMIA SYNDROMES

Disorder	Features	Diagnosis	Treatment

Acute Mesenteric Ischemia (AMI) - Arterial:	- acute abd pain out of proportion to physical findings
	- 75% with WBC > 15K, 50% with metabolic acidemia
	- "thumbprinting" on plain films of small bowel or R colon and → intestinal infarction
		1. selective mesenteric angiography mainstay
		2. CT to rule out other causes of sx
			1. treat precipitating cause
			2. Papaverine should not be used in pts in shock
			3. thrombolytic therapy if:
			  - partially occluding embolus
			  - embolus in branch of SMA or main SMA distal to ileocolic artery
			   and
			  - study performed within 24 hours of sx
			4. laparotomy prn, including second look 12–24 hours later

• superior mesenteric artery emboli (SAME)	- emboli usually from L atrial or ventricular mural thrombus - many patients with h/o previous peripheral emboli and 20% with synchronous emboli to other arteries		
• non-occlusive mesenteric (NOMI)	- results from splanchnic vasoconstriction from preceding cardiovascular event - ↑ risk with hemodialysis or major cardiac or intra-abdominal surgery - pain absent in 25%		

continued

• superior mesenteric artery thrombosis (SMAT)	- occur at areas of severe atherosclerotic narrowing, most often at origin of SMA - commonly superimposed on colonic ischemia (CI), with 20–50% with h/o intestinal angina - frequent h/o coronary, cerebral, or peripheral arterial ischemia	
Mesenteric Venous Thrombosis (MVT)	- seen in 5–10% of AMI cases - etiology: BCP, antithrombin III, protein S and C deficiency, polycythemia vera, myeloproliferative disorder		
• acute	- 20–50% mortality - abd pain initially out of proportion to physical findings, N&V and occult blood in 50%; gross GIB in 15% and → infarction, fever - duration of sx 1–2 wks before admission	1. CT scan diagnostic in 90%: - thickening and enhancement of bowel wall - enlarged superior mesenteric vein (SMV) w/ central lucency - dilated collateral vessels 2. selective mesenteric angiography	1. trial of heparin or thrombolytic therapy if no evidence of infarction 2. laparotomy if infarction present + heparinization × 7–10 d followed by Coumadin × 3 mos
• chronic	- asymptomatic or GIB usually from esophageal varices - physical findings of portal hypertension		

TABLE 29-11
INTESTINAL ISCHEMIA SYNDROMES (CONTINUED)

Disorder	Features	Diagnosis	Treatment
Focal Segmental Ischemia (FSI)	- etiology: atheromatous emboli, strangulated hernia, vasculitis, blunt abdominal trauma, XRT - usually adequate collateral circulation to avoid infarction - 3 presentations: 　1. acute enteritis - simulates appendicitis 　2. chronic enteritis - may simulate Crohn's disease 　3. obstruction - most common - may see "sentinel loop" or tapered stricture on imaging		Resection of involved bowel
Chronic Mesenteric Ischemia (CMI) - aka intestinal angina	- < 5% of cases of intestinal ischemia - almost always caused by mesenteric atherosclerosis - cardinal feature: meal-associated abd pain w/i 30 min w/ increasing severity and then gradual abatement over 1–3 h - expect to see food aversion and weight loss - abd bruit common	1. Doppler U/S, MRA, or spiral CT for screening 2. if screening test(s) abnormal, follow with splanchnic angiography: 　- usually see at least 2 of 3 splanchnic vessels either completely obstructed or severely stenosed	Revascularization procedure - surgery vs. angioplasty

| **Colon Ischemia (CI)** | - most common ischemic disorder of GI tract
- presentations:
 • reversible colopathy (~ 2/3)
 • transient colitis (~ 1/3)
 • perforation and gangrene
 • stricture
 • chronic segmental colitis
 • fulminant colitis
- may be confused with IBD or infectious colitis
- etiology: vasculitis esp SLE, sickle cell, coagulopathy, cocaine, long distance running, Rx - estrogen, NSAIDs; idiopathic in most cases
- sx: mild, LLQ pain, urge to defecate, bright red or maroon blood mixed with stool
- splenic flexure, descending colon, and sigmoid most common sites
- sx resolution usually 24–48 h and healing usually within 2 wks
- complication of aortic surgery in 1–7% of cases, as high as 60% of cases of aortic rupture, and responsible for 10% of deaths in aortic surgery
- obstructive lesion in 10–15% of cases: colon ca, stricture, diverticulitis, volvulus, fecal impaction, XRT stricture | Colonoscopy within 48 h of sx - hemorrhagic nodules with F/U exam 1 wk later which may show normal colon, evolution with segmental ulceration | 1. expectant:
- IVF
- abx
- optimization of cardiac fxn
- serial evaluation
2. laparotomy for infarction |

TABLE 29-12
DIFFERENTIATING FEATURES OF HEPATIC CANCER

Feature	Fibrolamellar ca	HCC
Age	23	55–60
Gender	male = female	male:female = 4:1
Cirrhosis	4%	80%
Cure rate	32%	0–34%
Survival	43 mos	6.5 mos

INDEX

A

Abdominal angina, 37*t*
Abetalipoproteinemia, 180
Abscess, hepatic, 130–132
  imaging of, 221
  treatment of, 134
Acalculous cholecystitis, 145–149
Acanthosis nigricans, 213
Acetaminophen
  drug reactions and, 118
  hepatotoxicity of, 122
Acetate
  deficiency and toxicity syndromes
    of, 270*t*
  sources and absorption site of, 200
Achalasia, 26, 27*f*, 28*f*, 30, 30*f*, 262*t*
Acid-peptic disease
  drug therapy for, 254*t*
  upper gastrointestinal bleeding in,
    70–71
Aciphex (pantoprazole), 254*t*
Acquired immunodeficiency syndrome
    (AIDS), 205–210, 206–209*t*, 210*f*
  gastrointestinal lymphoma and, 243
  hepatotoxicity of treatment for, 119*t*
Acromegaly, 274*t*
Acute cholecystitis, 147, 148
Acute diarrhea, 8*t*
Acute fatty liver of pregnancy, 176–178,
    258*t*
Acute gastritis, 228
Acute hepatic failure, 138
Acute hepatitis, 82
  diagnosis of, 92*t*
  laboratory features of, 91*t*
  during pregnancy, 259*t*
Acute hepatocellular necrosis, 89*t*
Acute intermittent porphyria, 111–112*t*
Acute mesenteric ischemia (AMI),
    35–42, 37*t*, 40*f*, 308*t*

Acute pancreatitis
  chromosomal changes in, 63
  computed tomography in, 159*f*
  demographics of, 154
  diagnostic tests for, 160–162*t*
  imaging in, 220
  Ranson criteria for, 166*t*
  signs and symptoms of, 155
  treatment of, 164
Acute porphyria, 110*t*, 114*t*
Adenocarcinoma
  colonic, 231
  gastric, 63, 64, 242
  small bowel, 242
Adenoma
  colonic, 231
  hepatic, 130, 131, 221, 232
  sebaceous, 213
  small bowel, 230
Aeromonas diarrhea, 11, 302*t*
  diagnosis of, 17
  signs and symptoms of, 15
  treatment of, 20, 22*t*
AIDS (acquired immunodeficiency syn-
    drome), 205–210, 206–209*t*, 210*f*
  gastrointestinal lymphoma and, 243
  hepatotoxicity of treatment for, 119*t*
Albendazole for *Microsporida*, 306*t*
Albumin, 184
  in hepatobiliary disorders, 89–90*t*
Alcoholic hepatitis, 232
  liver function tests in, 89*t*
  treatment of, 95
Alkaline phosphatase, 89–90*t*
Alpha$_1$–antitrypsin deficiency, 232, 278*t*
  demographics of, 123–124
  signs and symptoms of, 124
  treatment of, 127
Amebiasis, 231
Amebic hepatic abscess, 131

AMI (acute mesenteric ischemia), 35–42, 37*t*, 40*f*
Amino acids, 182
  in parenteral nutrition, 187–188
Aminolevulinic acid dehydrase deficiency, 111*t*, 114*t*
Aminotransferases, 89–90*t*
Amoxicillin, hepatotoxicity of, 122
Amoxicillin-clavulanic acid, 136
Ampicillin
  for *Listeria*, 298*t*
  for *Shigella*, 300*t*
Amylase, pancreatic, 160*t*, 181
Amylase/creatinine clearance ratio, 160*t*
Amyloidosis, 232
  Crohn's disease and, 57
  dermatologic manifestations of, 214
Anal cancer, 243
Anemia in Crohn's disease, 56
Angiodysplasia, 231
Angiography
  in hepatic mass, 219*t*
  pancreatic, 161*t*
Angiomyolipoma, 232
Angular stomatitis, 56
Annular pancreas, 224
Anthropometric measurements, 184
Anti-α4 antibody in inflammatory bowel disease, 60*t*
Antibiotics
  for *Campylobacter jejuni*, 298*t*
  for *Cyclospora cayetanensis*, 306*t*
  for *Escherichia coli*, 296*t*
  for infected ascites, 136
  for infectious diarrhea, 22*t*
  for inflammatory bowel disease, 59–61, 60*t*
  for *Isospora belli*, 306*t*
  for *Listeria*, 298*t*
  for prophylaxis in endoscopic procedures, 247
  for *Shigella*, 300*t*
  for *Vibrio cholera*, 296*t*
  for Whipple's disease, 304*t*
  for *Yersinia*, 301*t*
Antigen
  carcinoembryonic, 242*t*
  in hepatitis, 294–295*t*
Anti-*Helicobacter pylori* agents, 255*t*
Anti-hepatitis agents, 255–256*t*
Antiinflammatory agents, 254*t*
Antiviral therapy
  for hepatitis B, 97*t*
  for hepatitis C, 96*t*
  hepatotoxicity of treatment for HIV, 119*t*
Aphthous stomatitis, 56

Apolipoprotein B, 180
Arachidonic acid
  deficiency and toxicity syndromes of, 202, 270*t*
  sources and absorption site of, 199
Arteriovenous malformation, 71, 72, 73*t*
Arthropathy in inflammatory bowel disease, 55–56
Asacol (mesalamine), 254*t*
Ascites, 135–137, 136*t*
Ascitic fluid, 160*t*
Ascorbic acid
  deficiency of, 201, 268*t*
  dermatologic manifestations of deficiency or toxicity of, 214
  recommended dietary allowances of, 194*t*
  sources and absorption site of, 199
  toxicity of, 203, 268*t*
Attenuated familial adenomatous polyposis, 44
Autoimmune cholangiopathy, 281*t*
Autoimmune hemolytic anemia in Crohn's disease, 56
Autoimmune hepatitis, 232, 279*t*
  demographics of, 101
  diagnosis of, 103
  drug-related, 119
  laboratory features of, 93*t*
  signs and symptoms of, 102
  treatment of, 103–105, 104*t*
Autoimmune liver disease, 101–108, 107*t*, 279–281*t*
  demographics of, 101–102
  diagnosis of, 103
  signs and symptoms of, 102–103
  treatment of, 103–106, 104*f*, 104*t*, 105*t*
Avascular necrosis in Crohn's disease, 56
Azathioprine (Imuran), 103–104, 105*t*, 255*t*, 279*t*
Azulfidine (sulfasalazine), 254*t*

B
Bacillus cereus diarrhea, 9, 298*t*
  diagnosis of, 17
  signs and symptoms of, 14
  treatment of, 19
Bacterial diarrhea, 3, 296–304*t*
  demographics of, 7–12
  diagnosis of, 16–17
  empiric therapy for, 7
  inflammatory *versus* noninflammatory, 8*t*
  signs and symptoms of, 13–16
  treatment of, 19–21, 22*t*
Bacterial overgrowth, 6
Balantidium coli, 21, 307*t*

Bannayan-Ruvalcaba-Riley syndrome, 44, 284*t*
  signs and symptoms of, 47
  treatment of, 50
Bariatric surgery, 235–239
Barium enema in ulcerative colitis, 58
Barium imaging, 223–224
Barrett's esophagus, 227
  chromosomal changes in, 63
  surveillance protocols for, 241
Basal cell nevus syndrome, 45, 285*t*
Benign noncystic liver lesion, 129–132
Benign recurrent intrahepatic cholesta-
     sis, 135–137
Beriberi, 200, 266*t*
Bile acid diarrhea, 5, 11*t*
Bile salts, 179
Biliary cystadenoma, 221
Biliary tree, 145–149
  imaging of, 217–226, 224*f*
  pathology of, 232–234
Biliopancreatic diversion, 237
Bilirubin, 89–90*t*
Bioimpedance analysis, 184
Biopsy
  diagnostic impact of, 234
  hepatic, 233*f*
  small bowel, 229*t*, 234
Biotin
  deficiency of, 202, 270*t*
  recommended intakes of, 197*t*
  sources and absorption site of, 200
  toxicity of, 270*t*
Bismuth-tetracycline-metronidazole
     (Helidac), 255*t*
Blastocystis hominis, 21, 307*t*
Bleeding
  in diverticular disease, 75–77
  gastrointestinal, 69–74, 70*t*, 73*t*
  of obscure origin, 249
  in portal gastropathy, 137
Blind loop syndrome, 6
Bloody diarrhea, 6
Blue rubber bleb nevus syndrome, 214
Body mass index (BMI), 184, 235
Botox injection for achalasia, 262*t*
Bowel obstruction, 32
Budd-Chiari syndrome, 232
Butyrate
  deficiency and toxicity syndromes
     of, 270*t*
  sources and absorption site of, 200

C
Calcifications, pancreatic, 163*f*
Calcium
  absorption of, 182
  deficiency and toxicity syndromes
     of, 202, 271*t*
  recommended intakes of, 196*t*
Calculous disease, 145–149
Campylobacter jejuni diarrhea, 9, 298*t*
  in acquired immunodeficiency syn-
     drome, 209
  diagnosis of, 17
  signs and symptoms of, 14
  treatment of, 19, 22*t*
Cancer
  chromosomal changes in, 63
  colon, 43–52
    demographics of, 44–45
    gene alterations in, 46*t*
    risk factors for, 51*t*
    screening for, 48–49, 50*t*
    signs and symptoms of, 45–48
    treatment of, 49–50
  esophageal
    chromosomal changes in, 63
    surveillance protocols for, 241
    treatment regimens for, 242
  frequency of tumor metastasis to
     liver, 143*t*
  gallbladder, 146
  liver, 139–141
    demographics of, 143*t*
    differentiating features of, 312*t*
    imaging of, 140–142*f*
    liver function tests in, 90*t*
  pancreatic, 171*t*
    chromosomal changes in, 63
    demographics of, 155
    diagnostic tests for, 160–162*t*, 163
    endoscopic ultrasound of, 156*f*
    imaging in, 220, 221
    serologic markers in, 64
    signs and symptoms of, 157, 157*f*
    treatment of, 165, 242
  small bowel, 230
  surveillance protocols for, 241–245,
     242*t*
Candidal infection
  in acquired immunodeficiency syn-
     drome, 206*t*
  in diarrhea, 307*t*
  in esophagitis, 227, 248
Carbohydrates
  absorption of, 180–181
  in parenteral nutrition, 187
Carcinoembryonic antigen, 242*t*
Carcinoid, 228, 230, 275*t*
Carcinoid syndrome, 170–173, 171*t*
Carotene, deficiency and toxicity syn-
     dromes of, 203, 266*t*
Caustic ingestion, esophagus and, 248

Cefotaxime for infected ascites, 136
Celiac sprue, 229
    chromosomal changes in, 63
    dermatologic manifestations of, 214
    serologic markers in, 64
Cephalosporins for infected ascites, 136
Chest radiography in colon cancer sur-
        veillance, 242*t*
Child
    recommended dietary allowances
        for, 194–195*t*
    recommended intakes for, 196–197*t*
Cholangiocarcinoma, 139, 146–147, 220
Cholangitis, 147, 148, 218
Cholecystitis, 218
Choledochal cyst, 146–147, 221
Choledocholithiasis, 147, 148, 218
Cholelithiasis
    imaging in, 218, 222
    during pregnancy, 260*t*
Cholestasis
    benign recurrent intrahepatic,
        135–137
    drug-related, 119, 120–121*t*
    intrahepatic cholestasis of pregnancy
        and, 257*t*
    liver function tests in, 90*t*
Choline, 197*t*
Chromium
    deficiency and toxicity syndromes
        of, 198*t*, 201, 203, 270*t*
    sources and absorption site of,
        199
Chronic atrophic gastritis, 228
Chronic diarrhea, 9*t*
    diagnosis of, 18*f*
    traveler's, 6
Chronic gastritis, 228
Chronic hepatitis, 82
    antiviral therapy in, 96*t*, 97*t*
    laboratory features of, 91*f*, 93*t*
    liver function tests in, 89*t*
    during pregnancy, 259*t*
    signs and symptoms of, 85
Chronic mesenteric ischemia (CMI),
        35–42, 37*t*, 40*f*, 310*t*
Chronic pancreatitis
    demographics of, 154–155
    diagnostic tests for, 160–162*t*
    imaging in, 220
    signs and symptoms of, 155
    treatment of, 164–165
Chronic porphyria, 110–111*t*
Cimetidine (Tagamet), 254*t*
Ciprofloxacin
    for *Escherichia coli*, 296*t*
    for *Shigella*, 300*t*

Cirrhosis, 232
    ascites in, 135
    drug reactions in, 118
    liver function tests in, 89*t*
    nutritional support in, 189
    varices in, 137
Clostridium botulinum, 10, 15, 17, 20,
        302*t*
Clostridium difficile, 10, 15, 17, 301–302*t*
Clostridium perfringens, 10, 15, 17, 20,
        302*t*
CMI (chronic mesenteric ischemia),
        35–42, 37*t*, 40*f*, 310*t*
CMV (cytomegalovirus)
    in acquired immunodeficiency syn-
        drome, 206*t*, 208–209*t*
    in diarrhea, 13, 16, 17, 21, 305*t*
    in esophageal infection, 227
    in gastric infection, 228
    in liver disease, 233
Cobalamin
    deficiency and toxicity syndromes
        of, 200–203, 267–268*t*
    sources and absorption site of, 199
Colitis, 231
    in acquired immunodeficiency syn-
        drome, 209*t*
    diarrhea in, 6
    inflammatory, 4, 53–61
        diagnosis of, 57*t*, 57–58, 58*f*
        epidemiology of, 55*t*
        extraintestinal manifestations of,
            55–57
        signs and symptoms of, 53–55,
            54*t*
        treatment of, 58–61, 60*t*
    ischemic, 35–42
        diagnosis of, 38
        signs and symptoms of, 37*t*, 37–38
        treatment of, 39, 40*f*, 41*f*
    lower gastrointestinal bleeding in,
        72, 73*t*
Colitis cystica profunda, 224
Collagenous colitis, 231
Colon
    acquired immunodeficiency syn-
        drome and, 207–208*t*
    cancer of, 43–52, 282–287*t*
        chromosomal changes in, 63, 65*t*
        demographics of, 44–45
        gene alterations in, 46*t*
        lower gastrointestinal bleeding in,
            73*t*
        major syndromes in, 43–44
        risk factors for, 51*t*
        screening for, 48–49, 50*t*
        signs and symptoms of, 45–48

surveillance protocols for,
241–242, 242*t*
treatment of, 49–50, 243
idiopathic pseudo-obstruction of, 29
ischemia of, 35–42, 37*t*, 40*f*, 41*f*, 311*t*
motility disorders of, 31–33, 32*f*
pathology of, 230–232
Colonic diarrhea, 4, 10*t*, 14
Colonoscopy
in colon cancer surveillance,
241–242, 242*t*
in colon ischemia, 311*t*
in inflammatory bowel disease, 58
Computed tomography, 217–221
of hepatic mass, 219*t*
of hepatocellular carcinoma, 140*f*
pancreatic, 161*t*
Congenital erythropoietic porphyria,
114*t*
Copper
deficiency and toxicity syndromes
of, 198*t*, 201, 203, 269*t*
sources and absorption site of, 199
Cowden's syndrome, 44, 285*t*
dermatologic manifestations of, 214
screening for, 49
signs and symptoms of, 47
Crails syndrome, 44
Creon, 154*t*
CREST syndrome, 265*t*
Crohn's disease, 53–61, 228
diagnosis of, 57*t*, 57–58, 58*f*
epidemiology of, 55*t*
extraintestinal manifestations of,
55–57
nutritional support in, 189
signs and symptoms of, 53–55, 54*t*
treatment of, 59, 60*t*
Cronkhite-Canada syndrome, 45, 47,
232, 286*t*
dermatologic manifestations of, 214
Cryptosporidiosis, 13, 18, 230, 306*t*
in acquired immunodeficiency syndrome, 208*t*
signs and symptoms of, 16
treatment of, 22*t*
Cyclospora cayetanensis diarrhea, 13, 306*t*
in acquired immunodeficiency syndrome, 208*t*
signs and symptoms of, 16
treatment of, 21, 22*t*
Cyclosporine
drug reactions and, 118
toxicity of, 139
Cyst
choledochal, 146–147
hepatic, 130–134

pancreatic pseudocyst
demographics of, 155
diagnosis of, 163
signs and symptoms of, 156
treatment of, 165
Cystadenoma, 130, 132
Cystic fibrosis, 63
Cystic pancreatic tumor
demographics of, 155
diagnosis of, 163
signs and symptoms of, 156–157
treatment of, 165
Cytomegalovirus (CMV)
in acquired immunodeficiency syndrome, 206*t*, 208–209*t*
in diarrhea, 13, 16, 17, 21, 305*t*
in esophageal infection, 227
in gastric infection, 228
in liver disease, 233

D
Defecation disorders, 31–32
Delayed hypersensitivity skin testing,
184
Dermatologic manifestations
in Crohn's disease, 56
in gastrointestinal malignancy, 213
DES (diffuse esophageal spasm), 26, 30
Dextrose in parenteral nutrition, 187
Diabetes mellitus, diarrhea in, 5
Diarrhea, 3–23, 296–307*t*
in acquired immunodeficiency syndrome, 207*t*
acute, 8*t*
bacterial, 3, 296–304*t*
demographics of, 7–12
diagnosis of, 16–17
empiric therapy for, 7
signs and symptoms of, 13–16
treatment of, 19–21, 22*t*
bile acid *versus* fatty acid, 11*t*
carcinoid tumor and, 275*t*
chronic, 9*t*, 18*f*
diabetic, 5
drug-induced, 12*t*
fungal, 307*t*
inflammatory *versus* noninflammatory, 8*t*, 11*t*
microscopic colitis and, 6
oral rehydration therapy in, 181
parasitic, 4, 7, 13, 305–307*t*
signs and symptoms of, 18–19
treatment of, 21, 22*t*
secretory *versus* osmotic, 5*t*
small bowel *versus* colonic, 10*t*
traveler's, 6
VIPoma and, 273*t*

viral, 3–4, 13, 304–305*t*
    diagnosis of, 17
    signs and symptoms of, 16
    treatment of, 21
Diazoxide for insulinoma, 272*t*
Dietary fiber, 180
Dieulafoy's lesion, 71, 228
Diffuse esophageal spasm (DES), 26,
    30, 263*t*
Dipentum (olsalazine), 254*t*
Diuretics for cirrhotic ascites, 135
Diversion colitis, 231
Diverticular disease, 72, 75–77
Diverticulum, 231
Double duct sign of pancreatic cancer,
    157*f*
Drug therapy, 254–256*t*
    acute attack in porphyria and, 115*t*
    for *Campylobacter jejuni,* 298*t*
    hepatotoxicity of, 117–122
        HIV treatment and, 119*t*
        morphologic changes and,
            120–121*t*
        risk-factor associations in, 118–119
    for inflammatory bowel disease,
        59–61, 60*t*
    for *Listeria,* 298*t*
    for obesity, 236
    for *Shigella,* 300*t*
    for *Vibrio cholera,* 296*t*
    for *Yersinia,* 301*t*
Drug-induced diarrhea, 12*t*
Duodenal switch, 237–238
Duodenum, nutrient absorption in, 249
Dysplasia
    esophageal, 227
    gastric, 228
    in inflammatory bowel disease, 231

E
Echinococcus granulosus, 130
Eclampsia, 260–261*t*
Elemental formula, 186
Embolus, superior mesenteric artery, 36
Empiric therapy for diarrhea, 7
Encephalopathy, hepatic, 190
Endocrine syndromes, 169–173,
    272–275*t*
Endolimax nana, 307*t*
Endoscopic retrograde cholangiopan-
    creatography (ERCP), 162*t,*
    221–223, 224*f*
Endoscopic ultrasound, 218
    in pancreatic cancer, 156*f,* 162*t*
Endoscopy
    antibiotic prophylaxis for, 247
    in ulcerative colitis, 57–58, 58*f*

Entamoeba coli, 307*t*
Entamoeba hartmanni, 307*t*
Entamoeba histolytica, 13, 131, 306–307*t*
    signs and symptoms of, 16
    treatment of, 21, 22*t*
Enteral nutrition, 185–187
Enteric myopathy, 32, 32*f*
Enteric neuropathy, 32, 32*f*
Enterocolitis, 10
Enterohemorrhagic *Escherichia coli* diar-
    rhea, 8, 297*t*
    signs and symptoms of, 14
    treatment of, 19, 22*t*
Enteropathy in acquired immunodefi-
    ciency syndrome, 209*t*
Enteropeptidase, 181
Enterotoxigenic *Escherichia coli,* 297*t*
Eosinophilic gastritis, 228, 248
Episcleritis, 56
ERCP (endoscopic retrograde cholang-
    iopancreatography), 162*t,*
    221–223, 224*f*
Erythema multiforme, 56
Erythema nodosum, 56, 215*f*
Erythromycin for infectious diarrhea,
    22*t*
Erythropoietic porphyria, 113*t,* 114*t*
Escherichia coli diarrhea, 7–8,
    296–297*t*
    diagnosis of, 17
    signs and symptoms of, 13–14
    treatment of, 19, 22*t*
Esomeprazole (Nexium), 254*t*
Esophagitis desiccans, 227
Esophagus
    acquired immunodeficiency syn-
        drome and, 206*t*
    cancer of
        chromosomal changes in, 63
        surveillance protocols for, 241
        treatment regimens for, 242
    diffuse spasm of, 26, 30, 263*t*
    Mallory-Weiss tear and, 71
    motility disorders of, 25–30, 27*f,* 28*f,*
        30*f,* 31*f*
    nonspecific motor disorder of, 26, 29,
        30, 264*t*
    pathology of, 227
    pill esophagitis and, 247
Essential fatty acids
    deficiency and toxicity syndromes
        of, 202, 270*t*
    sources and absorption site of,
        199
Ethanol, drug reactions with, 118
Ethical considerations in nutritional
    support, 190–191

F

Familial adenomatous polyposis (FAP), 44, 282*t*
  chromosomal changes in, 63
  risk for colon cancer, 51*t*
  screening for, 48, 50*t*
  signs and symptoms of, 45
  surveillance protocols for, 242
  treatment of, 49
Famotidine (Pepcid), 254*t*
Fatty acid diarrhea, 11*t*
Fatty liver
  hepatotoxicity of drug therapy and, 120*t*
  imaging of, 221
Female
  recommended dietary allowances for, 194–195*t*
  recommended intakes for, 196–197*t*
FHF (fulminant hepatic failure), 98*t*
Fibrosis, drug-related, 119
Fish oil for inflammatory bowel disease, 60*t*
Fistula, pancreato-colic, 164*f*
Flat adenoma, 231
Fluoride, 196*t*
Flushing, 213
Focal nodular hyperplasia, 130, 232
  imaging in, 220–221
  signs and symptoms of, 131
Focal occult blood test, 241, 242*t*
Focal segmental ischemia (FSI), 35–42, 37*t*, 40*f*, 310*t*
Folate (folic acid)
  absorption of, 182–183
  deficiency of, 201, 268*t*
  dermatologic manifestations of deficiency of, 214
  recommended intakes of, 197*t*
  sources and absorption site of, 199
  for tropical sprue, 303*t*
  for Whipple's disease, 304*t*
Follicular gastritis, 228
Food poisoning, 8
Fructose, 181
FSI (focal segmental ischemia), 35–42, 37*t*, 40*f*, 310*t*
Fulminant hepatic failure (FHF), 98*t*, 138
Fundoplication, 249
Fungal diarrhea, 307*t*
Furosemide (Lasix), 135

G

Galactose, 181
Gallbladder cancer, 146
Gallstone ileus, 147, 148, 149

Gallstones, 147, 148
  imaging in, 218, 222
  during pregnancy, 260*t*
Gardner's syndrome, 44
  dermatologic manifestations of, 214
  surveillance protocols for, 242
Gastric adenocarcinoma
  chromosomal changes in, 63
  serologic markers in, 64
  treatment regimens for, 242
Gastric antral vascular ectasia (GAVE), 71, 228, 248
Gastric dysplasia, 228
Gastric erosion, 227
Gastric lymphoma, 242
Gastric ulcer, 228
Gastrinoma, 170–173, 272*t*
Gastroenteritis, 10
Gastrointestinal bleeding, 69–74
  dermatologic manifestations of, 214
  in diverticular disease, 75–77
  lower, 70*t*, 72–73, 73*t*
  upper, 70*t*, 70–71, 73*t*
Gastrointestinal stromal tumor (GIST), 222, 248
Gastrointestinal tract
  imaging of, 217–226, 219*t*, 222–224*f*
  pathology of, 227–234, 229*t*, 230*f*, 233*f*
Gastroparesis, 248
Gastropathy in acquired immunodeficiency syndrome, 207*t*
Gastroplasty, vertical banded, 236–237
GAVE (gastric antral vascular ectasia), 71, 228, 248
Gene alteration in colorectal cancer, 46*t*
Genetic liver disease, 123–127, 125*t*, 126*t*
Genetics, 63–67, 65*t*, 66*t*
Genitourinary disease, Crohn's disease and, 57
Giardia lamblia diarrhea, 13, 230, 305*t*
  diagnosis of, 18
  signs and symptoms of, 16
  treatment of, 21, 22*t*
Gilbert's syndrome, 89*t*
GIST (gastrointestinal stromal tumor), 222, 248
Glucagonoma, 170–173, 171*t*
Glucose, 181
Glycerin, 187
Glycerol, 187
Gorlin syndrome, 44, 47, 285*t*
Granuloma, drug-related, 121*t*
Granulomatous hepatitis, 119
Grehlin, 235–236
GRFoma, 170–173, 274*t*

H
Helicobacter pylori, 228, 255t
Helidac (bismuth-tetracycline-metroni-
    dazole), 255t
HELLP syndrome, 175–178, 176t,
    257–258t
Hemangioma
    hepatic, 129–130
    imaging of, 220, 222–223f
Hematologic disease, Crohn's disease
    and, 56
Hemobilia, 72–73
Hemochromatosis, 276t
    demographics of, 123
    diagnosis of, 124, 125t
    genetic testing for, 66t
    signs and symptoms of, 124
    treatment of, 126
Hemolysis
    liver function tests in, 89t
    in vitamin E deficiency, 266t
Hemorrhoids, 72, 73t
Hemosuccus pancreaticus, 72
Heparin
    for inflammatory bowel disease, 60t
    for mesenteric venous thrombosis,
        309t
Hepatic abscess, 130–132
    imaging of, 221
    treatment of, 134
Hepatic adenoma, 130
    imaging of, 221
    signs and symptoms of, 131
Hepatic encephalopathy, 190
Hepatic hemangioma, 129–131
Hepatic lymphoma, 243
Hepatic porphyrias, 109–115, 110–115t
Hepatic proteins, 184
Hepatitis, 288–295t
    antigens and antibodies in, 294–295t
    autoimmune, 232, 279t
    drug therapy for, 255–256t
    hepatotoxicity of drug therapy for,
        120–121t
    nutritional support in, 189
    during pregnancy, 259t
Hepatitis A, 288t
    antigens and antibodies in, 294t
    clinical and epidemiologic features
        of, 83–84t
    demographics of, 81
    diagnosis of, 85, 92t
    laboratory evaluation of, 87t
    signs and symptoms of, 82
    treatment of, 86
Hepatitis A vaccine, 86, 97t, 288t
Hepatitis B, 232, 288–290t

antigens and antibodies in,
    294–295t
antiviral therapy in, 97t
chronic, 93t
clinical and epidemiologic features
    of, 83–84t
demographics of, 81–82
diagnosis of, 86, 92t
drug therapy for, 255t
laboratory evaluation of, 87t, 91t
signs and symptoms of, 82–85
treatment of, 86, 92–93
Hepatitis B vaccine, 86, 97t, 288–289t
Hepatitis C, 232, 291–293t
    antigens and antibodies in, 295t
    clinical and epidemiologic features
        of, 83–84t
    demographics of, 82
    diagnosis of, 86, 92t
    drug therapy for, 255–256t
    indications and recommendations
        for antiviral therapy in, 96t
    laboratory evaluation of, 88t
    signs and symptoms of, 85
    treatment of, 93–95
Hepatitis D, 290–291t
    chronic, 93t
    clinical and epidemiologic features
        of, 83–84t
    demographics of, 82
    diagnosis of, 86
    treatment of, 95
Hepatitis E, 293t
    demographics of, 82
    diagnosis of, 86
    treatment of, 95
Hepatobiliary disorders, 89–90t
Hepatocellular adenoma, 232
Hepatocellular carcinoma (HCC), 130,
    232
    diagnosis of, 132
    differentiating features of, 312t
    imaging of, 140–142f
    liver transplantation in, 93
    paraneoplastic syndromes in, 139–141
    signs and symptoms of, 131
    treatment regimens for, 134, 243
Hepatopulmonary syndrome, 138
Hepatorenal syndrome (HRS), 137
Hepatotoxicity of drugs, 117–122
    HIV treatment and, 119t
    morphologic changes and, 120–121t
    risk-factor associations in, 118–119
Hereditary coproporphyria, 112t,
    114t
Hereditary hemorrhagic telangiectasia,
    214

Hereditary nonpolyposis colon cancer (HNPCC), 45, 286–287t
  chromosomal changes in, 63
  risk for colon cancer, 51t
  screening for, 49, 50t
  signs and symptoms of, 48
  surveillance protocols for, 242
  treatment of, 50
Herpes simplex virus (HSV)
  in acquired immunodeficiency syndrome, 206t, 209t
  in diarrhea, 13, 16, 17, 20, 305t
  in esophageal infection, 227
  in liver disease, 233
Hirschsprung's disease, 33
Histamine₂ blockers, 254t
Histoplasmosis, 307t
History and physical exam, 183–184
Hormones, obesity and, 235–236
Howel-Evans syndrome, 214
Human immunodeficiency virus (HIV), 205–210, 206t–209t, 210f
  gastrointestinal lymphoma and, 243
  hepatotoxicity of treatment for, 119t
Hydatid liver cyst, 130–134
Hyperemesis gravidarum, 175–178, 176t, 257t
Hyperplastic colon polyp, 231
Hyperplastic polyposis, 45, 48, 49
Hypertension after liver transplantation, 138
Hypertensive lower esophageal sphincter, 26, 29, 30, 263t
Hypertrichosis lanuginosa acquisita, 213
Hypertrophic gastric folds, 228

I

Idiopathic esophageal ulcer, 207t
Idiopathic intestinal pseudo-obstruction, 29, 265t
Immune globulin for hepatitis A, 86, 288t
Immunosuppressive antimetabolites, 255t
Imuran (azathioprine), 103–104, 105t, 255t, 279t
Inertia, colonic, 33
Infant
  recommended dietary allowances for, 194–195t
  recommended intakes for, 196–197t
Infected ascites, 135–136
Infection after liver transplantation, 139
Infectious diarrhea, 4, 6–7, 22t
Inflammatory bowel disease (IBD), 4, 53–61
  dermatologic manifestations of, 214

diagnosis of, 57t, 57–58, 58f
  drug therapy for, 254t, 255t
  dysplasia in, 231
  epidemiology of, 55t
  extraintestinal manifestations of, 55–57
  signs and symptoms of, 53–55, 54t
  surveillance protocols for, 242
  treatment of, 58–61, 60t
Inflammatory cloacogenic polyp, 232
Inflammatory diarrhea, 4, 8t, 9t, 11t
Infliximab (Remicade), 254t
Insulinoma, 169–173, 171t, 272t
Interferon alfa-2b (Intron A)
  for hepatitis B, 86, 92
  for hepatitis C, 94, 96t, 291–292t
  for hepatitis D, 290t
Interferon alfa-2b-ribavirin (Rebetron), 94, 96t, 292t
Interleukins for inflammatory bowel disease, 60t
Intestinal angina, 310t
Intestinal ischemia syndromes, 35–42, 308–311t
  diagnosis of, 38
  signs and symptoms of, 37t, 37–38
  treatment of, 39, 40f, 41f
Intrahepatic cholestasis of pregnancy, 175–178, 257t
Intrinsic neuropathy, 32
Intron A (interferon alfa-2b), 255t
Iodamoeba buetschii, 307t
Iodine
  deficiency and toxicity syndromes of, 202, 271t
  recommended dietary allowances of, 194t
  sources and absorption site of, 200
Iron
  absorption of, 182
  deficiency of, 183
  overload of, 66t, 232
  recommended dietary allowances of, 194t
Irritable bowel syndrome (IBS), 256t
Ischemia, intestinal, 38–39, 40f, 41f
Ischemic colitis, 35–42
  diagnosis of, 38
  signs and symptoms of, 37t, 37–38
  treatment of, 39, 40f, 41f
Ischemic liver disease, 232
Islet cell tumor, 222
Isoenzymes, pancreatic, 160t
Isoniazid, 118, 121
Isospora belli diarrhea, 13
  signs and symptoms of, 16
  treatment of, 21, 306t

J

Juvenile polyp, 231
Juvenile polyposis coli, 44, 284t
    screening for, 48–49
    signs and symptoms of, 47
    treatment of, 49

K

Kaposi's sarcoma, 207t, 210f, 214
Keshan's disease, 269t
Kidney stones, 57
Krukenberg's tumor, 214
Ku-Zyme HP, 154t

L

Lactation
    recommended dietary allowances
        during, 194–195t
    recommended intakes during,
        196–197t
Lamivudine for hepatitis B, 92–93, 290t
Lansoprazole (Prevacid), 254t
Lansoprazole-amoxicillin-clarithromy-
    cin (Prevpac), 255t
Laparoscopic adjustable gastric bands,
    237
Large bowel diarrhea, 4, 10t, 14
Lead intoxication, 114t
Leiomyosarcoma, 230
Leptin, 236
Leukocytosis in Crohn's disease, 56
Leuvocorin calcium, 306t
Linitis plastica, 222, 228
Linoleic acid
    deficiency and toxicity syndromes
        of, 202, 270t
    sources and absorption site of, 199
Linolenic acid
    deficiency and toxicity syndromes
        of, 202, 270t
    sources and absorption site of, 199
Lipid absorption, 179–180
Listeria diarrhea, 298t
Liver
    abscess of, 130–132
        imaging of, 221
        treatment of, 134
    acute fatty liver of pregnancy and,
        258t
    benign recurrent intrahepatic
        cholestasis and, 135–137, 136t
    frequency of tumor metastasis to, 143t
    imaging of, 217–226, 219t, 222–223f
    pathology of, 232–234
    portal gastropathy and, 137–138
    spontaneous rupture during preg-
        nancy, 261t

Liver cancer, 139–141
    demographics of, 143t
    differentiating features of, 312t
    imaging of, 140–142f
    liver function tests in, 90t
Liver disease
    biopsy in, 233f
    cystic, 130, 132–134
    dermatologic manifestations of,
        213–216, 215f
    genetic, 123–127, 125t, 126t
    hemochromatosis and, 276t
    nutritional support in, 189–190
    surgical considerations in, 129–134,
        133t
Liver failure, 138
Liver function tests, 89–90t, 242t
Liver transplantation
    in alpha₁–antitrypsin deficiency, 127
    in autoimmune hepatitis, 105, 279t
    in cirrhotic ascites, 135, 136
    complications of, 138–139
    in fulminant hepatic failure, 98t
    in hemochromatosis, 126
    in hepatitis B, 93, 290t
    in hepatitis C, 95, 293t
    in primary biliary cirrhosis, 105, 280t
    in primary sclerosing cholangitis,
        105–106, 281t
    rejection of, 139, 232
    in Wilson's disease, 277t
Long-chain triglycerides, 179
Lower esophageal sphincter
    achalasia and, 262t
    hypertensive, 26, 29, 30, 263t
    idiopathic intestinal pseudo-obstruc-
        tion and, 265t
Lower gastrointestinal bleeding, 69–74,
        70t, 73t
    in diverticular disease, 75–77
Lymphocytic colitis, 231
Lymphocytic gastritis, 228, 248
Lymphoma, 242–243
Lynch syndrome, 45, 286–287t
    screening for, 49
    signs and symptoms of, 48
    treatment of, 50

M

Macrocytic anemia, 200–201, 267–268t
Macrovesicular steatosis, 233
Magnesium
    deficiency and toxicity syndromes
        of, 202, 271t
    recommended intakes of, 196t
Magnetic resonance cholangiopancre-
        atography, 162t

Magnetic resonance imaging, 217–221
  of hepatic mass, 219*t*
  of hepatocellular carcinoma, 141*f*
Malabsorptive conditions
  chronic diarrhea and, 9*t*
  drug-induced diarrhea and, 12*t*
  small bowel biopsy in, 229*t*
Malabsorptive procedures, 237–238
Male
  recommended dietary allowances
    for, 194–195*t*
  recommended intakes for, 196–197*t*
Mallory bodies, 234
Mallory-Weiss tear, 71, 73*t*
MALT (mucosa-associated lymphoid
    tissue lymphoma), 228, 242
Manganese, deficiency and toxicity
    syndromes of, 198*t*, 201, 203,
    270*t*
Mass, hepatic, 219*t*
Meckel's diverticulum, 73
Medication-induced lesion, gastrointes-
    tinal bleeding in, 71
Medium-chain triglycerides, 180
Ménétrier's disease, 228, 248
6–Mercaptopurine, 255*t*
Mesalamine (Pentasa, Asacol, Rowasa),
    254*t*
Mesenteric venous thrombosis (MVT),
    35–42, 37*t*, 40*f*, 309*t*
Metabolic bone disease, 56
Metal deficiencies, 198*t*
Metastatic Crohn's disease, 56
Metastatic neuroendocrine tumors,
    275*t*
Metoclopramide (Reglan), 254*t*
Metronidazole
  for *Blastocystis hominis*, 307*t*
  for *Clostridium difficile* diarrhea, 301*t*
  for *Entamoeba histolytica*, 306*t*
  for *Giardia lamblia*, 305*t*
  for infectious diarrhea, 22*t*
  for toxic megacolon, 301*t*
Microscopic colitis, 6
Microsporidium diarrhea, 13, 18
  in acquired immunodeficiency syn-
    drome, 208*t*
  signs and symptoms of, 16
  treatment of, 21, 306*t*
Microvesicular steatosis, 233
Mid-arm circumference, 184
Mirizzi's syndrome, 145–149, 221
Molybdenum, deficiency and toxicity
    syndromes of, 201, 203, 270*t*
Monosaccharides, 181
Motility disorders, 25–33, 262–265*t*
  diarrhea and, 9*t*, 12*t*

drug therapy for, 254*t*
  motility study findings in, 26–29,
    27–31*f*
  small bowel and colonic, 31–33, 32*f*
  treatment of, 30
Mucosa-associated lymphoid tissue
    lymphoma (MALT), 228, 242
Muir-Torré syndrome, 45, 48, 214, 287*t*
Multiple endocrine neoplasia, 170, 275*t*
MVT (mesenteric venous thrombosis),
    35–42, 37*t*, 40*f*, 309*t*
Mycobacterium avium complex, 207*t*,
    209*t*

N
NASH (nonalcoholic steatohepatitis),
    63, 233
Nasoduodenal intubation, 186
Nasogastric intubation, 186
Necrosis, drug-related, 119, 121*t*
Neoplastic lesion, drug-related, 121
Nephrolithiasis, Crohn's disease and, 57
Neural tube defects, 268*t*
Neurofibromatosis, 214
Neurotransmitters, small bowel, 32
Nexium (esomeprazole), 254*t*
NHL (non-Hodgkin's lymphoma), 207*t*
Niacin
  deficiency of, 200, 267*t*
  recommended intakes of, 197*t*
  sources and absorption site of, 199
  toxicity of, 203, 267*t*
Nicotine for inflammatory bowel dis-
    ease, 60*t*
Nicotinic acid
  deficiency of, 200, 267*t*
  toxicity of, 203, 267*t*
NOMI (non-occlusive mesenteric
    ischemia), 36, 308*t*
Nonalcoholic steatohepatitis (NASH),
    63, 233
Non-cholera *Vibrio* diarrhea, 7, 296*t*
  diagnosis of, 17
  signs and symptoms of, 13
  treatment of, 19, 22*t*
Non-Hodgkin's lymphoma (NHL), 207*t*
Noninflammatory diarrhea, 4, 8*t*, 9*t*, 11*t*
Non-occlusive mesenteric ischemia
    (NOMI), 36, 308*t*
Nonspecific esophageal motor disor-
    der, 26, 29, 30, 264*t*
Nonsteroidal antiinflammatory drugs
    (NSAIDs), 248
Norfloxacin, 136
Norwalk agent, 13, 16, 17, 21, 305*t*
Nuclear medicine in hepatic mass, 219*t*
Nutcracker esophagus, 26, 29, 30, 263*t*

Nutrient absorption, 179–183
Nutrition, 179–191
    assessment of, 183–184
    calcium absorption and, 182
    carbohydrate absorption and,
        180–181
    Crohn's disease and, 189
    enteral, 185–187
    ethical considerations in nutritional
        support, 190–191
    folic acid absorption and, 182–183
    iron deficiency and, 183
    lipid absorption and, 179–180
    liver disease and, 189–190
    pancreatitis and, 188–189
    parenteral, 187–188
    protein absorption and, 181–182
    short bowel syndrome and, 190
    sulfasalazine-related folate defi-
        ciency and, 183
    vitamin B_{12} absorption and, 182, 183
Nutritional assessment, 183–184
Nutritional deficiencies, 193–204,
        266–271t
    dermatologic manifestations of,
        213–214
    metals and, 198t
    recommended dietary allowances
        and, 194–195t
    recommended dietary intakes and,
        196–197t
    sources and absorption sites of nutri-
        ents and, 199–200
    toxicity syndromes and, 202–203t
    of vitamins, 200–202t

O
Obesity, bariatric surgery for, 235–239
Obstructive uropathy, Crohn's disease
        and, 57
Occult gastrointestinal hemorrhage, 72
Octreotide
    for glucagonoma, 273t
    for VIPoma, 272t
Ofloxacin, 136
Olsalazine (Dipentum), 254t
Omega-3 fatty acids for inflammatory
        bowel disease, 60t
Omeprazole (Prilosec), 254t, 272t
1307K APC gene mutation, 44, 48, 283t
Ophthalmologic disease in Crohn's dis-
        ease, 56
Oral rehydration therapy, 181
Orlistat, 236
Oroduodenal intubation, 186
Orogastric intubation, 186
Orthotopic liver transplantation, 138–143

Osler-Weber-Rendu disease, 214
Osmotic diarrhea, 5t
    chronic, 9t
    drug-induced, 12t
Osteomalacia, 56
Osteopenia, 56
Osteoporosis, 56
Overlap syndrome, 101–108, 107t, 281t
    demographics of, 102
    signs and symptoms of, 103
    treatment of, 106

P
Paget's disease, 214
Pancrease, 154t
Pancreatic amylase, 181
Pancreatic cancer, 171t
    chromosomal changes in, 63
    demographics of, 155
    diagnostic tests for, 160–162t, 163
    endoscopic ultrasound of, 156f
    imaging in, 220, 221
    serologic markers in, 64
    signs and symptoms of, 157, 157f
    treatment of, 165, 242
Pancreatic cholera, 171t
Pancreatic enzymes
    for steatorrhea, 154t
    in testing for pancreatic disorders,
        160–161t
Pancreatic lymphoma, 243
Pancreatic pathology, 234
Pancreatic polypeptide, 161t
Pancreatic proteases, 181
Pancreatic pseudocyst
    demographics of, 155
    diagnosis of, 163
    signs and symptoms of, 156
    treatment of, 165
Pancreatitis
    acute
        chromosomal changes in, 63
        computed tomography in, 159f
        demographics of, 154
        diagnostic tests for, 160–162t
        imaging in, 220
        Ranson criteria for, 166t
        signs and symptoms of, 155
        treatment of, 164
    chromosomal changes in, 63
    chronic
        demographics of, 154–155
        diagnostic tests for, 160–162t
        imaging in, 220
        signs and symptoms of, 155
        treatment of, 164–165
    nutritional support in, 188–189

Pancreato-colic fistula, 164f
Pancrelipase, 154t
Pantoprazole (Aciphex), 254t
Pantothenic acid, 197t
Paracentesis for cirrhotic ascites, 135
Paracoccidioidomycosis, 307t
Paraneoplastic syndromes, 139–141
Parasitic diarrhea, 4, 7, 13
    diagnosis of, 18–19
    inflammatory *versus* noninflamma-
        tory, 8t
    signs and symptoms of, 16
    treatment of, 21, 22t
Parenteral nutrition, 187–188
PBC (primary biliary cirrhosis),
        101–108, 107t
Peginterferon alfa-2b for hepatitis C, 94,
        256t, 293t
Peliosis hepatis, 232
Pellagra, 200, 267t
Pelvic floor dyssynergia, 33
Penicillamine for Wilson's disease,
        126t, 127
Pentasa (mesalamine), 254t
Pepcid (famotidine), 254t
Peptic ulcer disease
    drug therapy for, 254t
    upper gastrointestinal bleeding in,
        70–71, 73t
Peptidases, 182
Percutaneous endoscopic gastrostomy
        (PEG), 186
Percutaneous endoscopic gastrostomy
        with jejunal extension (PEGJ),
        186
Peripheral parenteral nutrition (PPN),
        188
Pernicious anemia, 183
Peutz-Jeghers syndrome, 44, 231, 283t
    dermatologic manifestations of, 214
    screening for, 48
    signs and symptoms of, 45–47
    treatment of, 49
Phenytoin, hepatotoxicity of, 122
Phlebotomy in hemochromatosis, 126
Phospholipidosis, drug-related, 119
Phosphorus
    deficiency and toxicity syndromes
        of, 202, 271t
    recommended intakes of, 196t
Physical examination, 183–184
Pill esophagitis, 247
Pituitary adenoma, 275t
Plain films, 223–224
Plesiomonas diarrhea, 11, 302–303t
    diagnosis of, 17
    signs and symptoms of, 15

    treatment of, 20, 22t
Pleural fluid studies, 160t
Plummer-Vinson disease, 214
Pneumatosis intestinalis, 223–224, 231
Polycystic liver disease, 130
    diagnosis and treatment of, 132
    imaging in, 221
Polymeric formula, 185
Polyp, biliary, 146–147
Polypharmacy, 119
Polyposis, 43–52, 282–287t
    demographics of, 44–45
    dermatologic manifestations of, 214
    risk for colon cancer, 51t
    screening for, 48–49, 50t
    signs and symptoms of, 45–48
    treatment of, 49–50
Porcelain gallbladder, 224
Porphyria cutanea tarda, 113t, 114t
Porphyrias, 109–115, 110–115t
Portal gastropathy, 137–138
Postinflammatory colon polyp, 232
Potassium, deficiency and toxicity syn-
        dromes of, 202, 271t
Prealbumin, 184
Prednisone for autoimmune hepatitis,
        103–104, 105t, 279t
Preeclampsia, 177, 260–261t
Pregnancy, 257–261t
    acute fatty liver of, 258t
    acute viral hepatitis in, 259t
    cholelithiasis in, 260t
    chronic viral hepatitis in, 259t
    HELLP syndrome in, 175–178, 176t,
        257–258t
    hyperemesis gravidarum in,
        175–178, 176t, 257t
    intrahepatic cholestasis of, 175, 177,
        257t
    preeclampsia and eclampsia in,
        260–261t
    recommended dietary allowances in,
        194–195t
    recommended intakes during,
        196–197t
    spontaneous hepatic rupture in, 261t
    Wilson's disease in, 260t
Prevacid (lansoprazole), 254t
Prevpac (lansoprazole-amoxicillin-
        clarithromycin), 255t
Prilosec (omeprazole), 254t, 272t
Primary biliary cirrhosis (PBC),
        101–108, 107t, 232, 280–281t
    demographics of, 101
    diagnosis of, 103
    signs and symptoms of, 102–103
    treatment of, 105

Primary sclerosing cholangitis (PSC),
      101–108, 107*t*, 232, 281*t*
   chromosomal changes in, 63
   demographics of, 101–102
   diagnosis of, 103
   endoscopic retrograde cholangio-
      pancreatography, 224*f*
   imaging in, 220
   signs and symptoms of, 103
   treatment of, 105–106
Pro-kinetic/pro-motility agents, 254*t*
Prophylaxis for endoscopic procedures,
      247
Propionate
   deficiency and toxicity syndromes
      of, 270*t*
   sources and absorption site of, 200
Protein
   absorption of, 181–182
   in parenteral nutrition, 187–188
   recommended dietary allowances of,
      194*t*
   restriction in hepatic encephalopa-
      thy, 190
Prothrombin time in hepatobiliary dis-
      orders, 89–90*t*
Proton-pump inhibitors, 254*t*, 272*t*
Protoporphyria, 114*t*
Pruritus in intrahepatic cholestasis of
      pregnancy, 177
PSC (primary sclerosing cholangitis),
      101–108, 107*t*
Pseudocyst, pancreatic
   demographics of, 155
   diagnosis of, 163
   signs and symptoms of, 156
   treatment of, 165
Pseudomembranous colitis, 231
Psoriasis, 56
Pyoderma gangrenosum, 56
Pyogenic hepatic abscess, 130
Pyridoxine
   deficiency of, 200, 267*t*
   sources and absorption site of, 199
   toxicity of, 203, 267*t*
Pyrimethamine for *Isospora belli,* 306*t*

Q

Quinacrine for *Giardia lamblia,* 305
Quinolones for infectious diarrhea,
      22*t*

R

Radiation colitis, 231
Ranitidine (Zantac), 254*t*
Ranitidine-bismuth (Tritec), 255*t*
Ranson-Imrie criteria, 158*f,* 166*t*

Rebetron (interferon alfa-2b-ribavirin),
      94, 96*t*, 255*t*, 292*t*
Recommended dietary allowances,
      194–195*t*
Recommended dietary intakes,
      196–197*t*
Rectal cancer
   gene alterations in, 46*t*, 65*t*
   treatment regimens for, 243
Recurrent diarrheal syndrome, 20
Recurrent pyogenic cholangitis,
      145–149
Reflux esophagitis, 227
Reglan (metoclopramide), 254*t*
Rejection of liver transplantation, 139,
      232
Remicade (infliximab), 254*t*
Renal insufficiency after liver trans-
      plantation, 138
Resection of small bowel, 249
Retinol
   deficiency of, 200, 266*t*
   dermatologic manifestations of defi-
      ciency or toxicity of, 213
   recommended dietary allowances of,
      194*t*
   sources and absorption site of, 199
   toxicity of, 202, 266*t*
Retinol-binding protein, 184
Rheumatologic disease, dermatologic
      manifestations of, 214
Ribavirin-interferon for hepatitis C, 94
Riboflavin
   deficiency of, 200, 267*t*
   dermatologic manifestations of defi-
      ciency or toxicity of, 213
   recommended intakes of, 197*t*
   sources and absorption site of, 199
   toxicity of, 203, 267*t*
Rickets, 271*t*
Rotaviral diarrhea, 13, 16, 17, 21, 304*t*
Roux-en-Y gastric bypass, 238
Rowasa (mesalamine), 254*t*

S

Sacroiliitis in Crohn's disease, 56
Salmonella typhi diarrhea, 10, 299*t*
   in acquired immunodeficiency syn-
      drome, 209*t*
   diagnosis of, 17
   signs and symptoms of, 14
   treatment of, 19, 22*t*
SAME (superior mesenteric artery
      emboli), 36, 308*t*
Schwachman-Diamond syndrome, 64
Scintigraphy, 217
Scleroderma

acral sclerosis and digital ulcers in, 29f
CREST syndrome and, 265t
dermatologic manifestations of, 214
esophageal motility and, 26, 29, 30
Screening
for colon cancer, 48–49, 50t
for Cowden's syndrome, 285t
for juvenile polyposis coli, 284t
for Lynch syndrome, 286–287t
for Peutz-Jeghers syndrome, 283t
Scurvy, 201, 268–269t
Sebaceous adenoma, 213
Secretin-cholecystokinin test, 162t
Secretory diarrhea, 5t
chronic, 9t
drug-induced, 12t
Selective angiography, pancreatic, 161t
Selenium
deficiency of, 198t, 201, 269t
recommended dietary allowances of, 194t
sources and absorption site of, 199
toxicity of, 198t, 203, 269t
Semi-elemental formula, 185–186
Serologic markers, 64, 92t
Serotonin receptor antagonist, 256t
Serum amylase, 160t
Serum lipase, 160t
Serum trypsinogen, 160t
Shigellosis, 10, 231, 300t
in acquired immunodeficiency syndrome, 209t
diagnosis of, 17
signs and symptoms of, 14–15
treatment of, 19–20, 22t
Short bowel syndrome, 190
Short-chain fatty acids
deficiency and toxicity syndromes of, 270t
sources and absorption site of, 200
Sibutramine, 236
Sigmoidoscopy, 242t
Sister Mary Joseph's nodule, 214
Skin
Crohn's disease and, 56
gastrointestinal malignancy and, 213
liver disease and, 213–216, 215f
Skin testing, delayed hypersensitivity, 184
Small bowel
acquired immunodeficiency syndrome and, 207–208t
adenocarcinoma of, 242
biopsy of, 229t, 234
lymphoma of, 63, 242
motility disorders of, 31–33, 32f

pathology of, 228–230, 230f
resection of, 249
Small bowel diarrhea, 4, 10t, 13–14
Small cell lung cancer, 64
SMAT (superior mesenteric artery thrombosis), 36
Snow White sign, 250
Sodium
absorption of, 181
deficiency and toxicity syndromes of, 202, 271t
Sodium-glucose co-transporter, 181
Solitary juvenile polyposis syndrome, 44, 47, 283t
Solitary rectal ulcer syndrome (SRUS), 231
Somatostatinoma, 170–173, 171t, 274t
South American blastomycosis, 307t
Spirochetosis, 231
Spironolactone for cirrhotic ascites, 135
Spondylitis in Crohn's disease, 56
Spontaneous hepatic rupture, 261t
Staphylococcus aureus diarrhea, 8, 298t
diagnosis of, 17
signs and symptoms of, 14
treatment of, 19
Steatorrhea, 180
in bacterial overgrowth, 6
pancreatic enzymes for, 154t
Steatosis, 233
drug-related, 119
Stent obstruction, 221
Stomach
acquired immunodeficiency syndrome and, 207t
cancer and, 63
pathology of, 227–228
Stress-related mucosal injury, 248
Sulfadiazine for *Isospora belli*, 306t
Sulfasalazine (Azulfidine), 254t
folate deficiency and, 183
Superior mesenteric artery emboli (SAME), 36, 308t
Superior mesenteric artery thrombosis (SMAT), 36, 309t
Surgery in liver disease, 129–134, 133t
Surveillance protocols for malignancy, 241–245, 242t
Swallowing difficulty, 26, 27f, 28f, 30, 30f, 262t
Sweet's syndrome, 56

T
Tacrolimus toxicity, 139
Tagamet (cimetidine), 254t
Tegaserod maleate (Zelnorm), 256t

Tetracycline
    for infectious diarrhea, 22*t*
    for tropical sprue, 303*t*
    for *Vibrio cholera,* 296*t*
Thalidomide for inflammatory bowel
        disease, 60*t*
Thiamine
    deficiency of, 200, 266–267*t*
    recommended intakes of, 196*t*
    sources and absorption site of, 199
    toxicity of, 203, 266–267*t*
Thrombocytosis in Crohn's disease, 56
Thromboembolism, Crohn's disease
        and, 56
Thrombosis
    mesenteric venous, 35–42, 37*t*, 40*f*
    superior mesenteric artery, 36
Tocopherol
    deficiency of, 200, 266*t*
    recommended dietary allowances of,
        194*t*
    sources and absorption site of, 199
    toxicity of, 202, 266*t*
Total lymphocyte count, 184
Total parenteral nutrition (TPN), 188
Toxic megacolon, 20, 54–55, 301*t*
Toxic porphyria, 114*t*
Toxicity syndromes, 202–203*t*
    dermatologic manifestations of,
        213–214
Transferrin, 184
Traveler's diarrhea, 6
Triceps skinfold measurement, 184
Trientine for Wilson's disease, 126*t*
Triglycerides, 180
Trimethoprim-sulfamethoxazole (TMP-
        SMX)
    for *Cyclospora cayetanensis,* 306*t*
    for *Escherichia coli,* 296*t*
    for infectious diarrhea, 22*t*
    for *Isospora belli,* 306*t*
    for *Listeria,* 298*t*
    for *Shigella,* 300*t*
    for Whipple's disease, 304*t*
Triphasic helical computed tomogra-
        phy of hepatic mass, 219*t*
Tritec (ranitidine-bismuth), 255*t*
Tropheryma whippelii, 12, 304*t*
    diagnosis of, 17
    signs and symptoms of, 15–16
    treatment of, 20–21
Tropical sprue, 11–12, 303*t*
    diagnosis of, 17
    signs and symptoms of, 15
    treatment of, 20
Trousseau's syndrome, 214
Trypsin, 181–182

Tuberculosis, 228, 303*t*
    in acquired immunodeficiency syn-
        drome, 207*t*
    diagnosis of, 17
Tubular adenoma, 231
Tumor
    in acquired immunodeficiency syn-
        drome, 207*t*
    biliary, 145–149
    frequency of metastasis to liver, 143*t*
    gastrointestinal stromal, 248
    pancreatic, 171*t*
        demographics of, 155
        diagnostic tests for, 160–162*t*, 163
        endoscopic ultrasound of, 156*f*
        signs and symptoms of, 157, 157*f*
        treatment of, 165
Turcot's syndrome, 44, 45, 287*t*
Tylosis palmaris, 213
Typhoid fever, 10, 14

U
Ulcerative colitis, 53–61, 230–231
    diagnosis of, 57*t*, 57–58, 58*f*
    epidemiology of, 55*t*
    extraintestinal manifestations of,
        55–57
    signs and symptoms of, 53–55, 54*t*
    treatment of, 58–59, 60*t*
Ultrase, 154*t*
Ultrasound, 218–221
    of hepatic mass, 219*t*
    of hepatocellular carcinoma, 140*f*
    pancreatic, 161*t*
Upper gastrointestinal bleeding, 69–74,
        70*t*, 73*t*
Upper gastrointestinal radiography,
        161*t*
Urine amylase, 160*t*
Uveitis in Crohn's disease, 56

V
Vaccine
    hepatitis A, 86, 97*t*, 288*t*
    hepatitis B, 86, 97*t*, 288–289*t*
Vancomycin for *Clostridium difficile*
        diarrhea, 301*t*
Varices, 71, 73*t*, 137
Variegate porphyria, 112*t*, 114*t*
Vascular lesion
    drug-related, 121
    upper gastrointestinal bleeding in,
        71
Verner-Morrison's syndrome, 272–273*t*
Vertical banded gastroplasty, 236–237
Vibrio cholera, 7, 296*t*
    diagnosis of, 16–17

signs and symptoms of, 13
  treatment of, 19, 22*t*
Vibrio parahaemolyticus, 7, 296*t*
  diagnosis of, 17
  signs and symptoms of, 13
  treatment of, 19
Vigorous achalasia, 26, 30, 262–263*t*
Villous adenoma, 231
Viokase, 154*t*
VIPoma, 170–173, 272*t*
Viral diarrhea, 3–4, 13, 304–305*t*
  diagnosis of, 17
  inflammatory *versus* noninflamma-
      tory, 8*t*
  signs and symptoms of, 16
  treatment of, 21
Viral hepatitis, 81–99, 288–295*t*
  antigens and antibodies in, 294–295*t*
  antiviral therapy in, 96*t*, 97*t*
  demographics of, 81–82, 83–84*t*
  diagnosis of, 85–86
  laboratory evaluation of, 87–88*t*
  liver function tests in, 89–90*t*
  liver transplantation in fulminant
      hepatic failure, 98*t*
  during pregnancy, 259*t*
  signs and symptoms of, 82–85
  treatment of, 86–95
  vaccination in, 97*t*
Virchow's node, 213
Vitamin A
  deficiency of, 200, 266*t*
  dermatologic manifestations of defi-
      ciency or toxicity of, 213
  recommended dietary allowances of,
      194*t*
  sources and absorption site of, 199
  toxicity of, 202, 266*t*
Vitamin B_1
  deficiency of, 200, 266–267*t*
  sources and absorption site of, 199
  toxicity of, 203, 266–267*t*
Vitamin B_2
  deficiency of, 200, 267*t*
  dermatologic manifestations of defi-
      ciency or toxicity of, 213
  sources and absorption site of, 199
  toxicity of, 203, 267*t*
Vitamin B_3
  deficiency of, 267*t*
  sources and absorption site of, 199
  toxicity of, 200, 203, 267*t*
Vitamin B_6
  deficiency of, 267*t*
  recommended intakes of, 197*t*
  sources and absorption site of, 199
  toxicity of, 200, 203, 267*t*

Vitamin B_{12}
  absorption of, 182, 183
  deficiency of, 267–268*t*
  sources and absorption site of, 199
  toxicity of, 200, 203, 267–268*t*
Vitamin C
  deficiency of, 201, 268*t*
  dermatologic manifestations of defi-
      ciency or toxicity of, 214
  recommended dietary allowances of,
      194*t*
  sources and absorption site of, 199
  toxicity of, 203, 268*t*
Vitamin D
  deficiency of, 202, 271*t*
  recommended intakes of, 196*t*
  sources and absorption site of, 200
  toxicity of, 271*t*
Vitamin deficiencies, 193–204, 266–271*t*
  dermatologic manifestations of,
      213–214
  recommended dietary allowances
      and, 194–195*t*
  recommended dietary intakes and,
      196–197*t*
  sources and absorption sites of nutri-
      ents and, 199–200
  toxicity syndromes and, 202–203*t*
Vitamin E
  deficiency of, 200, 266*t*
  recommended dietary allowances of,
      194*t*
  sources and absorption site of, 199
  toxicity of, 200, 202, 266*t*
Vitamin K
  deficiency of, 200, 266*t*
  recommended dietary allowances of,
      194*t*
  sources and absorption site of,
      199
  toxicity of, 200, 203, 266*t*

W
Water, absorption of, 181
Wernicke-Korsakoff encephalopathy,
    267*t*
Wet beriberi, 200, 266*t*
Whipple's disease, 12, 229, 304*t*
  diagnosis of, 17
  histopathology of, 230*f*
  signs and symptoms of, 15–16
  treatment of, 20–21
Wilson's disease, 277*t*
  demographics of, 123
  diagnosis of, 124–125
  liver biopsy in, 233*f*
  during pregnancy, 260*t*

signs and symptoms of, 124
treatment of, 126*t*, 127

X
Xanthelasma, 228

Y
Yersinia diarrhea, 10, 300–301*t*
diagnosis of, 17
signs and symptoms of, 15
treatment of, 20, 22*t*

Z
Zantac (ranitidine), 254*t*

Zelnorm (tegaserod maleate), 256*t*
Zinc
deficiency of, 198*t*, 201, 268–269*t*
dermatologic manifestations of deficiency or toxicity of, 214
recommended dietary allowances of,
194*t*
sources and absorption site of, 199
toxicity of, 198*t*, 203, 268–269*t*
Zinc salts for Wilson's disease, 126*t*
Zollinger-Ellison's syndrome (ZES),
171*t*, 228, 272*t*
drug therapy for, 254*t*
steatorrhea in, 180